To my Favorite Reader,

Vu-Preston Young

05/03

The Naked Chiropractor

Insider's Guide To Combating Quackery And Winning The War Against Pain

Dr. Preston H. Long

Introduction *by* Dale Dauten

Edited *by* Peter J. Weber

Cover Art *by* Robin Fox & Associates

First Printing, 2002

ISBN 0-9722816-0-6

Published by Evidence-Based Health Services, Inc.

2421 East Southern Avenue - Suite 5 - Tempe, Arizona 85282 - (480) 540-3264

The Naked Chiropractor

Insider's Guide To Combating Quackery And Winning The War Against Pain

Dr. Preston H. Long

Introduction *by* **Dale Dauten**

Edited *by* **Peter J. Weber**

Cover Art *by* **Robin Fox & Associates**

First Printing, 2002

ISBN 0-9722816-0-6
Library of Congress Control Number 2002093490

Published by **Evidence-Based Health Services, Inc.**
2421 East Southern Avenue - Suite 5 ~ Tempe, Arizona 85282 - (480) 540-3264
Visit us online at www.ebhs-inc.com

Contents

Contents 1

Acknowledgments 5

Introduction 6

Chapter 1

Welcome to the World of Chiropractic Care 9
- Test Your Chiropractic I. Q. 11
- Top Ten Signs You've Gone to a Bad Chiropractor 13
- Test Your Chiropractic I. Q. Answers 14

Chapter 2

The Making of a Chiropractor 16
- The School and Requirements 18
- Student Loans 19
- Meet The Students 20
- My First Adjustment 22
- Getting Started 22
- Jury Awards $285,019 to Former Cleveland Chiropractic College Students 23
- Not the First Lawsuit 25
- Julie Bernet Affidavit 25
- School's Out, Self-Employed and On My Own 29

Chapter 3

My Change of Life 32
- Independent Medical Examinations 33
- Stories That Speak for Themselves! 34

Chapter 4

From the Offbeat to the Fraudulent 37
- When A Chiropractic Adjustment Is Not What You Need 39
- Pediatric Chiropractic Care Lures More Believers 41
- Veterinary Chiropractic 45
- State Board of Chiropractic Examiners 46
- Why Won't Your State Board of Chiropractic Protect You? 47
- When Is A Doctor Not A Doctor? 48
- Sucking In Patients 48
- Perpetuating Fraud 49
- Attention All Auto Accident Victims 51
- More Actual Fraud Cases 52

Chapter 5

Hope For Those In Pain 54
- Face-to-Face With Your Mortality, How Will You React? 61
- Ah, The Key Word: Acceptance 62

Chapter 6

Deciding Where To Take Your Pain........64
Indications For Traditional Care........67
Is Physical Therapy The Solution?........67

Chapter 7

Alternative Medicine Is Encroaching on The Back Pain Business........70
Acupuncture: The Sticking Point of Alternative Medicine........70
Can Herbs Help?........73
Homeopathy: If A Lot Is Bad, A Little Is Better........73
Naturopathy: The Science of One-Stop Shopping........74
IOC Bans Austrians in Blood Transfusion Case........76
Will Simple Bed Rest Help?........76
Good Health Will Take a Small Effort from You........77
Ortho or Neuro Specialist?........77

Chapter 8

Selecting A Chiropractor Who Can Help You, Not Bankrupt You........80
Rule 1: Get Off The Mis-Information Superhighway........80
Rule 2: Know What Professional Memberships Are and What They Mean to You 82
Rule 3: Know The Two Main Types of Chiropractors........83
Rule 4: Look to Those With Experience........84
The Key Point Is... 87
Rule 5: Watch Your Wallet........88
Making Your Appointment........88
Rule 6: Insist on Full Disclosure........90
Rule 7: Bring a Healthy Dose of Skepticism........94
Remember These Additional "Don'ts"........95
Is Chiropractic Against Your Religion?........97
Rule 8: Protect Yourself – The Exam........98
The X-Factor: X-rays ... A Very Real Danger........100
...Free To Administer Any Therapy They Wish – Or Can Get Away With!........100

Chapter 9

The Kindly Giant's Guide to Back Care........101
Do Not Let This Happen To You!........101
Do-It-Yourself Treatments – A Guide To ... Inexpensive Symptom Control........103
Time For Special Attention - Exercises........104
If Pain Persists, Then Manipulation Is Not The Answer........111
P-A-I-N-E-D........113

Understanding Acute Low Back Problems........115
About the Back and Back Problems........115
Causes of Low Back Problems........116
Things To Do About Low Back Problems........117
Getting Relief........120
Proven Treatments........120
Other Treatments........121
Physical Activity........122
Bed Rest........122
About Work and Family........122
Things You Can Do Now........123

If You Are Not Getting Better 124
About Surgery 124
Prevention of Low Back Problems 125
When Low Back Symptoms Return 125
While Your Back is Getting Better 125

Chapter 10

My Opinion Is The Only One That Counts And Other Ironies of Alternative Medicine 127
The Opposite Viewpoint 129
The Myth of Whiplash 133
Science and Truth vs. Quackery and Greed 135
Evidence-based Medicine - EBM - Defined 136
Thoughts on Evidence-Based Medicine 137

CHAPTER 11

My Future for Chiropractic 139
The Education 139
Paradigm Shift 141
Self-Imposed Regulation 142

Appendix A

Useful Resources 145
Acute Low Back Pain in Adults: Assessment and Treatment 145

Table 1. Red Flags For Potentially Serious Conditions 148
Medical History 148
Physical Examination 149
Addressing Red Flags 149
Observation and Regional Back Examination 149
Neurologic Screening 149
Testing for Muscle Strength 150
Reflexes 151
Sensory Examination 151
Clinical Tests For Sciatic Tension 151
Initial Care 154
Patient Education 154
Patient Comfort 154
Oral Pharmaceuticals 155

Table 2. Symptom Control Methods 155
Physical Methods 155
Activity Alteration 156

Table 3. Guidelines For Sitting And Unassisted Lifting 158
Special Studies and Diagnostic Considerations 158
Selection of Special Studies 159

Table 4. Ability of Different Techniques 161
Management Considerations After Special Studies 161
Surgical Considerations 161
Direct And Indirect Nerve Root Decompression For Herniated Discs 163
Management of Spinal Stenosis 163

Table 5. Summary of Guideline Recommendations 166
Availability of Guidelines 166

Appendix B

References and Recommended Reading 168
Internet Sites 168
Books 168
Articles 169

Appendix C

Glossary 172

Appendix D

State Boards of Chiropractic Examiners 181

Appendix E

Chiropractic Colleges & Universities 187

Appendix F

Additional References 189

Notable Quotes 197
Index 198

Acknowledgments

A lot of people behind the scenes have made this book possible. First and foremost, I want to thank my wife, Eileen and my children, Caitlin and P. Alexander. Their patience and love especially during some very trying and stressful times in my career mean the world to me.

I also want to thank author Dale Dauten. I appreciate him for his insistence that I write this book and his emphasizing that it needed to be written by someone with an insider's perspective on chiropractic. I most appreciate "The Gifted Boss" for his friendship.

I want also to express appreciation to Debra, who swayed but never broke under my persistence and timelines. The hours of conversations and this new friendship are valued.

I offer a note of hope for the future: that the chiropractic profession will grow out of its dependence on specious claims and realize what it can legitimately provide to patients with relief and help them return to active living.

I also want to acknowledge you, the back pain sufferer, for whom this book is dedicated.

Introduction

By Dale Dauten

When the late Speaker of the House Tip O'Neill would run into someone he recognized but whose name he could not remember, he would ask, **"How is your back?"** The cagey old congressman knew that just about everyone had back troubles, so instead of being the dumb brick who forgot names, he was instead the amazing guy who remembered and sympathized.

Why did that question work so reliably for O'Neill? Sure, eighty percent of the population will have back problems in their lives, but an even higher percentage will have colds or the flu or other ailments. You would not ask, "How is your cold?" No, colds go away. Back problems seem to never leave. It seems you do not "get over" back problems ... you just have good days and bad days.

That is how it was for me for a decade or more, until 1995. It was with little hope for relief that I dragged my aching back to the office of Dr. Preston Long. I had seen two M.D.s and a chiropractor already, given up tennis and basketball, changed mattresses and office chairs. I went to Long as a favor to my wife, who was, I suppose, tired of watching me pretend I was not in pain.

Long looked at some x-rays I had brought along, felt along my spine, then, to my bafflement, pronounced it healthy. The problem, he told me, was chronic muscle spasms. As I came to understand what was going on, it was a single muscle gone mad, sending out frantic signals to the nervous system, like one of those car alarms set off by mistake. He hooked up a muscle stimulation device that made the muscle contract until it was exhausted and agreed to relax. Next he gave me some exercises and sent me home. **No "therapy plan" or follow-up.** just, "Do the exercises and if the pain still bothers you, come back." He added, "Don't worry – we will get you back on the tennis courts."

Months later, long after I had forgotten about doing back exercises, the car-alarm of a pain went off again and I returned to Long's office. There, while the muscle stimulation machine did its job, I pestered Long about his career and work. I write newspaper columns about work and business, and had written about medical practice previously, so I was curious on several levels. Why had two physicians failed to help me?

Why had the previous chiropractor I had visited wanted to see me three times a week forever? One said, "Let's do the three times a week for a few months and then we will re-evaluate. After all, your spine has spent years getting out of alignment. It is going to take a while to get it back where it should be."

As I talked with Long, on that day and on many other days as we became friends, I had an unpleasant realization: curing back problems is a tough way to make a living. **It is much more profitable to see one patient fifty times than it is to find fifty patients and cure them in one visit.**

Because of what he does and the sort of man that he is, Long is often hired as a consultant by insurance companies to review claims. He has served as an expert witness in many trials, arbitrations and depositions. And so he gets to see more of his profession than he would care to. For instance, one chiropractor charged a patient's insurance company for treatments made while the patient in question happened to be in Europe. The doctor explained that he had taken a photograph of the patient's aura, and continued to do "**aura adjustments**" using the photo while the patients were abroad.

Another case involved a woman who was sitting in front of a grocery store in her Buick Park Avenue when an empty shopping cart rolled off the curb and bumped her car. The car was not damaged, but she sought out a lawyer. The lawyer sent her to a chiropractor who prescribed a series of treatments. Long was hired to give his expert opinion on the effects upon of the human spine of an empty shopping cart bumping a Park Avenue.

My favorite of Long's tales from the courtroom is of the chiropractor who listed his diagnosis on the insurance forms as "**bruised karma.**"[1] I loved that diagnosis because I think it describes the state of medical care in this country.

We have a system where patients do not trust doctors, who do not trust insurance companies, who do not trust anyone. And who can blame them ~ any of them? The "health care debate" of the early 1990s has turned into the "health care 'resigned sigh'." It is a national case of bruised karma.

As I came to know and admire Preston Long, I urged him to write a book that might just help heal our karma.

---

[1] Except from "Medical System Needs A Healthy Debate" by Dale Dauten; *The Arizona Republic*, Section E, page 4; November 25, 1996. See also: Appendix.

As for my own back, I wish that Tip O'Neill were around and would ask me about it. I would say, "It feels great. Let's play some tennis."

****

Let me introduce Preston Long...

...AT SIX FEET, EIGHT INCHES, 280 POUNDS, DR. LONG literally fills a doorway. He is a man of such goodwill and ready humor that when I first wrote about him I described him as a “kindly giant.” Many of his patients saw the article, and turned that description into a nickname. And so, I step aside and give you over to the Kindly Giant, Dr. Preston Long, who comes to you fully clothed, but ready to bare the secrets of his profession, good and bad.

Chapter 1

Welcome to the World of Chiropractic Care

I wore a neck brace for about a year. It wasn't an accident or anything, I just got tired of holding my head up.

--Margaret Smith

In all likelihood, you will be among the eight out of every ten Americans who will suffer from back pain at some point. Worldwide, back pain is common. More treatments are touted for back pain than any other medical condition. As this book is written for you, the medical consumer, the goal is to shine a light on scientific evidence based on the most current clinical research, and do so in an easy to understand format.

In my years as a chiropractor and a consultant reviewing the various treatments rendered by health care providers, I came to realize that most providers have little or no understanding of back pain or how to make it go away inexpensively and easily. It is also clear that patients do not know how to help themselves, which they can do with ease. Sufferers have little or no understanding primarily due to lack of education from health care providers.

In the mid-1990s, I began fighting to decrease treatment variation and increase the use of evidence-based medicine. It has been an uphill battle. Let me share the details of this battle by focusing in on the chiropractic industry—the practice of chiropractic and chiropractic treatments, generally. In chiropractic, more than 400 techniques are used to treat acute back pain. If chiropractic is so wonderful and so perfect according to its believers, why do chiropractors treat only ten percent of the nation's population? And, in other nations, the percentage of patients treated is far lower—perhaps only one or two percent. In some countries, there are no chiropractors at all, or chiropractic is not permitted. Here is why Chiropractors have a problem: at the root, the vast majority of their techniques have no scientific foundation.

Of the 326 books about back pain currently in print, most contain far more opinion, belief, and testimonials than science. That is because back pain is not a science. The treatment of it can be.

In a vast majority of cases, back pain is a temporary condition. But that does not stop thousands of alternative medicine practitioners from trying to treat your back pain at considerable expense to you. As you will discover in the pages of this book, alternative medicine practitioners are very adept at patient solicitation and at "educating" them on a particular technique – and most of all, engendering patient satisfaction. The benefits patients experience from alternative medicine derive more from the way a treatment is presented than from the treatment itself. From an alternative medicine provider's point of view, getting you to accept convoluted logic and believe in the value of your treatment is nearly half the battle in resolving your problem.

Consumers need an advocate, someone who is not touting herbs, supplements, treatment modalities that you must pay someone else to perform, or even the expense of a gym membership. A true advocate does not try to gloss over the situation and tell you that you can cure pain by purchasing this system or this set of treatments. A true advocate reminds you that – while the power to make your pain go away is within you – if it does not, then it is not your fault.

That is not what complementary and alternative medicine providers do. There is a short name for complementary and alternative medicine: CAM. A CAM provider may tell you that you have the resources within you to make pain go away, but they will claim those resources only work in conjunction with their particular remedy. They will say their remedy is the key to unlocking your innate ability to heal yourself. We have a ripe environment for fraud and abuse, because back pain is usually more severe than other types of pain. People with back pain are often willing to try anything, believe anything, accept any recommendation. If a chiropractor says what you need are thirty "adjustments, spinal manipulations" or to "crack your back," then the severity of your pain may prompt you to nod in agreement.

Most of us have our "war stories" of bad chiropractic experiences. Chiropractic has been around for over one-hundred years, prompting us to wonder "where did it go wrong?"

I received my chiropractic education in Missouri, the "Show Me" state. Yet in my classroom, "Don't Show Me" ~ i.e. confuse me, hide logical thought, sway me with rhetoric, not facts- ~ was the order of the day. If you think that I am hinting that many of the problems are rooted in the teaching/learning processes, give yourself an "A" grade.

We will devote a chapter to the education of chiropractors. For now we can make a major point by saying that Chiropractors resist evidence-based medicine because, for them, actual science is not profitable. Pseudo-science is, however. And pseudo-science is the foundation for every chiropractor who has ever been in practice anywhere in the world. Some realize it; most do not. If you do, give yourself another "A" grade.

The chiropractic practitioners who still passionately embrace what they learned in their training have not escaped the dark cave of chiropractic theosophy. They want to keep you in the cave with them.

To assist you from ever entering this cave, let us examine the depth of your chiropractic knowledge. Following is a Chiropractic I.Q. Test asking ten questions relating to historical and contemporary chiropractic. Remember that the higher the score, the less distance you will travel into "mother chiropractic" and the dark cave of its theosophy. A score of eight or higher and you will probably pass by the cave with the mildest of interest and the least chance of being a patient for life. A score of five to eight, you will enter the cave smelling the moss on the walls, but beware as you will experience the enticement of traveling deep into the abyss. Any score below five and you are probably, unless you heed the information in this book, going to join the cave members forever.

Go ahead. Take the test. Good luck. After you read *The Naked Chiropractor* book, I suggest you return to this Chiropractic I.Q. Test and breeze through it a second time. Hopefully, the folly of your initial wrong answers can be washed away forever.

Test Your Chiropractic I. Q.

1) Visiting a chiropractor for an adjustment in an attempt to alleviate neck pain and/or stiffness and/or headaches can lead to a stroke or even death.

   True or False?

2) Chiropractic was founded by a magnetic healer/grocer whose claims have never been duplicated

   True or False?

3) Chiropractors treat a range of patients from newborn infants to horses?

True or False?

4) Chiropractors must earn a undergraduate degree prior to be accepted to a chiropractic College.

True or False?

5) Chiropractors have the highest amount of defaulted student loans of any professionals.

True or False?

6) Acute back pain will resolve on its own, without treatment by a chiropractor, 85-95% of the time.

True or False?

7) Generally, chiropractors employ consistent treatment techniques for same or similar conditions.

True or False?

8) Chiropractors are involved in Medicare and Veterans affairs.

True or False?

9) Chiropractors can be called the legislative profession.

True or False?

10) Chiropractors are trained to detect and correct subluxations.

True or False?

Before we see how you did, let us have some comic relief with another list of "Ten." What follows is a classic David Lettermen's Top Ten List! You may have seen or heard this before; in addition to television, a slightly watered-down version appeared in a chiropractic college newspaper.

—— David Letterman's Top Ten List[2] ——

Top Ten Signs You've Gone to a Bad Chiropractor

#10 WHEN YOU WALK, YOU MAKE A WACKY ACCORDION SOUND

#9 KEEPS SAYING, "A SPINE IS LIKE A BOX OF CHOCOLATES."

#8 REPEATEDLY ASKS, "YOU A COP? YOU SURE YOU AIN'T NO COP?"

#7 OVER AND OVER, YOU HEAR CRUNCHING SOUNDS FOLLOWED BY "UH-OH"

#6 THERE IS A TWO DRINK MINIMUM

#5 AT THE END SESSION, LIES DOWN ON THE TABLE AND SAYS, "MY TURN!"

#4 HE WAS NO WHERE NEAR WOODSTOCK AND YET HE'S COVERED WITH MUD

#3 RUSHES IN LATE FOR APPOINTMENT, STILL WEARING HIS BURGER KING UNIFORM

#2 HINTS THAT FOR AN EXTRA FIFTY BUCKS, HE'LL "STRAIGHTEN" SOMETHING ELSE

#1 YOU'RE FULLY CLOTHED AND HE'S NAKED

A couple more items have been added to the list – what follows were found in a chiropractic college newsletter [3]:

#11 WEEKS LATER, YOU SEE A GUY ON THE STREET SELLING VIDEOS OF YOUR VISIT

---

[2] -- "Top Ten List", *Late Night With David Letterman;* (1994, August 18)

[3] from "David Letterman's Top Ten List" (1999, April). *The Synapse*, p. 12.

#12 HE THROWS IN A COMPLIMENTARY RABIES SHOT

#13 WHILE MAKING ADJUSTMENT, HE PRETENDS TO PULL A SILVER DOLLAR OUT OF YOUR BUTT

#14 SPENDS HOURS PUSHING TOY CARS UP AND DOWN YOU BACK MAKING 'VROOM' SOUNDS

#15 YOU HAVE TO PUSH ASIDE DIRTY DINNER PLATES IN ORDER TO LIE DOWN ON THE EXAMINATION TABLE

Test Your Chiropractic I. Q.
ANSWERS

1. ***Deadly TRUE!*** As more consumers are lured to try alternative medical philosophies, such as chiropractic, more and more data becomes available on topics like death and stroke. In 1996 a Danish study analyzed a decade of data and concluded that one in every 120,00 neck manipulations resulted in stroke. In 1999, the Canadian Stroke Consortium, after studying data from fifteen stroke centers, concluded that one in every 100,00 chiropractic patients under 45 years of age will suffer a stroke after going to a chiropractor for neck problems. However, one the largest United States malpractice carriers for chiropractors has never produced any information on the subject.

2. ***Scientifically TRUE!*** The first chiropractic treatment has never been duplicated in 106 years. It was reported to cure a man's hearing in 1895. Using chiropractic techniques to cure a hearing problem has not happened since.

3. ***Amazingly TRUE!*** Newborns and animals are the fastest growing segments to be targeted. "Advanced" degrees can be gotten during weekend seminars. Stories are proudly reported of adjustments being given to newborns with the umbilical cord still attached, and an adjustment to the horse the infant may ride in a few years.

4. ***Academically FALSE!*** As of 2002 only one chiropractic college requires a bachelors degree for admittance. The other colleges only require sixty hours at a 2.0-2.5 GPA.

5. ***Financially TRUE!*** Chiropractors receive only 9% of original HEAL funding but greater than 50% of loan defaults are committed by chiropractors. Latest figures exceed 77 million dollars of defaulted chiropractic student loans.

6. ***Naturally TRUE!*** The natural history of a strain or simple mechanical acute back pain is that it will improve without treatment 85-95% of the time. The good news is it will happen in less than six weeks. The US Department of Health and Human Services state that if spinal manipulation does not work within four weeks, then that spinal manipulation should be stopped.

7. ***Unfortunately FALSE!*** There are over 200-400 "techniques" that chiropractors will use to attempt to treat your back. For every chiropractor there is almost as many philosophies available to explain your bad back. Techniques range from spring loaded clicky-looking guns to treating x-rays (not the patient – the patient's x-rays) to questioning your body for vitamin deficiencies.

8. ***Sadly TRUE!*** Chiropractic lobbying efforts have fought for inclusion in Medicare and most recently Veteran hospitals. In 2002, President George W. Bush signed into law chiropractic inclusion into Veteran hospitals.

9. ***Believe it, it is TRUE!*** As seen in Answer #8 above, the profession is on the legislative move. Many chiropractic major victories have been bought at the political level. This is, of course, because they have nothing to offer at the scientific level.

10. ***Consistently TRUE!*** Whether you have heard of subluxations or not, the chiropractic subluxation is the foundation of the profession and has been for 106 years. Unfortunately for chiropractors everywhere, subluxations have never been proven to exist. During all this time, the profession has never agreed upon a definition or at what level a subluxation needs to exist to cause health problems. Would you like to know what a subluxation is, really? A lot of people would, and so would I. That aside, no studies have been published that consumers who receive chiropractic care live longer and with less health concerns than people who do not.

Chapter 2

The Making of a Chiropractor

Lotta self-help tapes out there. Got one called 'How to Handle Disappointment.' I got it home and the box was empty.

--Jonathan Droll

"Oh, Honey, are you SURE?"

That was my mother's first reaction to my announcement that I was going to attend chiropractic college. My father added, "Have you really thought this through?" The tense questioning was my parents' Midwestern way of saying, "Are you CRAZY?" They asked the same question they would have asked if I had announced instead that I was joining the circus.

But that changed the following week. When my mother confided to the family accountant that her son was throwing away his future on becoming a chiropractor, the accountant surprised her, saying the tax statements of chiropractors showed that some of them made "serious money." The average income for chiropractors in the U.S. in 1981 was over $80,000. That was enough to open my parents' minds.

It was the Summer of 1981 and I had just graduated from college with a B.A. in Biology. My choice of a major had come from working as an orthopedic technician for Columbia Hospital in Milwaukee. But neither my work experience nor my education had induced me to undertake any serious career analysis. So, like many young graduates, my desire to continue my education was fueled by one simple reality: I did not know what else to do.

As I began to picture myself in various jobs, I started to eliminate possibilities. I did not have the patience or money to pursue medical school. I had been accepted into the cytotechnology program at the University of Wisconsin-Madison, using electron microscopes for blood research, but I knew myself well enough to know that I needed a people-person job. And I also knew that to be happy I needed to end up self-employed.

Then I read about chiropractic. Helping. Healing. Good money. Self-employed. I had never been to a chiropractor, but then I had never been to a mortician or a cytotechnician, either. I took the list of chiropractic colleges and called the first one: Cleveland Chiropractic College. They were good salespeople ~ after a few minutes on the telephone, I soon had a destination, a graduate school, a career.

I find it more than slightly ironic that I attended chiropractic college in the "Show Me" state of Missouri. From my very first week as a student at Cleveland Chiropractic College in Kansas City, I was demanding evidence for the absurd, outrageous contentions espoused by the president of the college and my teachers.

During that eye-opening first week the president of the college taught a "philosophy" class. In the cave of chiropractic, "philosophy" ~ or religious "theosophy" as it is more correctly called ~ can run the gamut from "subluxations cause every ailment imaginable" to "chiropractors are qualified to practice virtually every form of complementary and alternative medicine." During his weeks of lectures, he seemed to lean more toward the "subluxation theory." Singling me out during a lecture, he suggested that the reason I did not have allergies but my then-new wife did was that she had subluxations. Huh? I wondered, since when does the spine influence the way the bronchial tubes react to irritants or allergens? It did not make anatomical sense to me, and it should not. So, as for being loyal to the chiropractic brotherhood, I knew I was in trouble from the start.

People have asked me, "Why didn't you just quit right then and there?"

Today, with the wisdom that comes with age, I would have. At that point, I was 25, newly married, and not brave enough to say, "Oops, I made a big mistake." And, in my naiveté, I kept thinking to myself, "This is a school for health care practitioners. It cannot be as ridiculous as it seems right now." And, I was determined to be self-employed in my career. This path would give me that opportunity.

In the weeks and months that followed I became more and more disillusioned. There was a total lack of consensus among the "clinicians." The "professors" all taught different techniques for every symptom presented or discussed. Each teacher had his own favorite "hammer," as in, "when all you have in your toolbox is a hammer, every problem becomes a nail." Ouch! The

ubiquitous theory in much of alternative medicine is that every problem can be fixed with a single regimen. Of course, there is no agreement about what that regimen should be, because there are precious few or no clinical studies to support the claim that "xyz treatment" is the cure for whatever ails you, and that is a fact.

The School and Requirements

Education is the ability to listen to almost anything without losing your temper or your self-confidence.

--Robert Frost

Despite the name, Cleveland Chiropractic College is located in Kansas City, Missouri. My first sight of it was a crashing disappointment. Not only was it in a questionable neighborhood, it was smaller than my grammar school. A rambling building, undistinguished, set in the midst of a neighborhood that seemed scary, and was.

My fellow future chiropractors were a mixed lot. New students entered each trimester, about forty at a time. To my knowledge, no one flunked out. If you failed courses, you simply retook them. Some were professionals looking for a new start. One was a pharmacist, for instance. Most were quite young. You do not need a college degree to enter chiropractor college, at least not in most states. What is required is some basic college course prerequisites. So, we had twenty-year-olds and forty-year olds.

The admission requirements to enter chiropractic college are probably not what you think. In 2002 only one college requires a bachelors degree, the other seventeen or so do not. The typical requirements for admission are sixty hours of classes with a 2.5 GPA. That is approximately two years of college with a C grade point average. In fact, a C or 2.0 is all that is required in the basic science courses such as Biology and Chemistry.

Once a student is accepted, at least in one chiropractic college, the chances are excellent they can teach after graduation at their alma mater. "*Hiring your own*" has never been a practice widely accepted in the academic world, but this ~ remember ~ is the chiropractic world. A chiropractic college in Georgia lists in its 2000-2001 student catalog approximately 272 faculty members, of that number 143 are graduates of the institution, 34 are chiropractors from other colleges. This adds up to a grand total of 177 chiropractors teaching other chiropractors. Just think of the "*new ideas*" these students are exposed to everyday.

The majority of chiropractic colleges over the years have been owned and operated by old chiropractic families. They consider themselves as proud pioneers, handing down the schools from generation to generation.

Student Loans

These colleges do not receive public funding and are almost 100% dependent on student loans to remain open for business. Not to be obvious, but I hope you see the picture that is beginning to form. For colleges to remain open they are dependent on student loans to pay faculty, so a 2.0 GPA is all that is required for admission into these institutions of higher education. The more students who make the grade, the more loans can be applied for, right?

Outside of guaranteed student loans the other major source of the colleges income is from the HEAL loan program. HEAL stands for Health Education Assistance Loan. Here is a revealing statistic: HEAL funds only 9% of chiropractic-but over 50% of all HEAL loan defaults are by chiropractors. If you are interested to see if your chiropractor or just the one down the street made the default list, go to www.defaulteddocs.dhhs.gov. Remember the college that routinely hires their own as instructors? Lets see how they do as an institution in defaulted student loans from its graduates. You may have guessed it by now, they are #1, at $20,320,468.00 – *twenty million dollars*. So much for academic inbreeding!

Since you asked, here are the defaulted student loan figures for all the professions in the mid-1990s.

Allopathic Medicine including M.D.s	*$21,585,970*
Chiropractic	*$77,499,271*
Clinical Psychology	*$3,130,817*
Dentistry	*$41,281,154*

Health Administration	*$ 294,792*
Optometry	*$2,655,085*
Osteopathy	*$5,854,157*
Pharmacy	*$1,446,570*
Podiatry	*$20,077,616*
Public Health	*$603,934*
Veterinary Medicine	*$ 33,674*

Total Student Loan Defaults ~
HEAL Loan Program Only: ***$174,463,040!***

Meet The Students

There was no typical chiropractic student in my class or college but there were some interesting individuals to say the least. The most colorful of my classmates was a guy who looked like a character from the movie *Easy Rider*. He was rough looking piece of work, arriving each morning on his Harley, a bandanna over his head. He was able to attend class thanks to a "work-release program" that allows inmates to leave incarceration during the day to work or attend school, then return to spend nights back in jail.

Another classmate was a brilliant young man with a master's degree in philosophy. He was also a hard-core alcoholic. Devoted to jogging, on his runs he would take with him a water bottle filled with vodka. Prior to attending classes each morning, he would down a tumbler of vodka.

Perhaps the best way to sum up the quality of my fellow students is to say that, of the forty who entered with me, I trusted only two to perform medical procedures on me. Sadly, this was no academic conjecture but an awful reality, for we practiced on one another, even drawing each other's blood and giving rectal or breast exams. It should be mentioned that the limitations placed on chiropractors vary from state to state. In some places chiropractors can do blood work and even deliver babies. In others, they are limited to little more than manipulation.

Spinal manipulation ~ or chiropractic adjustment – is the main treatment option for chiropractors. You know: the old "crack your back" approach to health care. It is similar to cracking your knuckles. The chiropractor, places their hands (hopefully not some other part of their body) on the patient, and through some sort of technique, cures the patient, or gives a yank, makes a noise, or causes some pain.

As for the education itself, because I had worked in labs and hospitals, and had studied biology, I thought I understood the principles of science. I was unprepared for the philosophy of some of the instructors, which seemed more related to faith than science. The basic tenet of that faith was "subluxation" ~ the technical term for the bone out-of-place concept. Much of what passed for science was little more than the accumulation of anecdotes. A common storyline went something like this: a chiropractor would treat a patient for a back problem and her insomnia ~ or rash or indigestion or cancer ~ also went away. Such stories have become ingrained in what could be described as sort of chiro-cultural folk wisdom.

> ***I hope you recall the story of mine, asking the president of the college for his thoughts on why my wife had allergies and I did not. His response, expressed reasonably, was that the bones in my wife's upper thoracic region were out of place while mine were not. With my a priori understanding of allergens, antigens, and the human immune system, this made no sense to me. But, wanting an "A" and not a "C-" I bit my tongue, hoping that it would all be made clear, later, somehow. It never was made clear.***

Few of my classmates doubted the basic premise of spinal manipulation as the key to health. These new true believers could not wait to start saving the world one spine at a time. One classmate boasted that he had given an adjustment to his newborn son while the umbilical cord was still attached. Another attempted to treat his wife, only to put her in the hospital with torticollis. That is where the neck locks in place, tilted to one side.

We heard healing stories of every variety. One of those stories is the reason that I stayed on at Cleveland Chiropractic despite being surrounded by shaky science and shady characters. I pressed on for one simple reason, because of one healing story: my own.

My First Adjustment

I had had back problems all my life. My back "went out" many times, usually resulting in six to eight weeks of agony. At six-foot-eight, I had come to believe that I would always be vulnerable to this debilitating pain. I once spent two weeks in traction in college. And when I worked for a group of surgeons, I saw how little relief they had to offer. So I accepted my agony spells as inevitable. I was not surprised when, three months into my time at Cleveland Chiropractic, my back went out. One of the interns offered his help. He adjusted my lower back that day, a Thursday, then again on Friday. Before the weekend was over, I was fine. This was the identical problem that I had lived in fear of, knowing it meant two months of limping agony, now healed in just days. Here was a healing gift that I could share with the world.

And so I soldiered on at Cleveland Chiropractic College. I completed “school” and graduated after the standard three years. My fellow graduates tended to believe that they were superior to M.D.s, that they replaced the risks of drug therapies and surgeries with the ability to get the body to heal itself. My own beliefs were more modest: I felt I was ready to help people get rid of back pain.

Getting Started

To open a business is very easy; to keep it open is very difficult.

-- Chinese Proverb

One of the basic assumptions of our education at Cleveland Chiropractic College was that getting patients was not a problem. We were told that public interest in chiropractic was mushrooming, and why not? We could cure just about anything with some simple spinal adjustments. So, we believed that if we opened an office, people would start seeking out our services. This is known as the "build it and they will come approach.”

This was not the result in 1981-1984 when I was in school. Classmates opened their shops, then waiting and waited. From one year to the next, the waiting never improved.

The problems with Chiropractic schools are many, but the magnet for lawsuits is that students do NOT receive the education that had been promised by the colleges. Ultimately, there will be lawsuits over the validity of chiropractic itself. A disgruntled student or field chiropractor will bring the following lawsuit in some version: the individual will sue the chiropractic profession for taking their money and years of their life. The reason? Breach of contract, fraud, misrepresentation. The chiropractic organizations, schools, or practitioners will be sued because they accepted money and time from individuals, yet returned nothing. You are taught to diagnose, detect, monitor, and treat something that does not exist.

Listed below is an affidavit and other information relating to two separate instances where my college was sued. Note the various reasons why.

In 1999, fifteen 1997 graduates of Cleveland Chiropractic College of Kansas City, Missouri filed a lawsuit charging that my alma mater had failed to provide adequate teaching as promised by promotional literature and school representatives [1]. The suit sought a total of $22 million for breach of contract, unjust enrichment, and fraud. A local headline read:

Jury Awards $285,019 to Former Cleveland Chiropractic College Students

The allegations included:

- During the recruiting process, school representatives said that the clinical experience they would receive would be invaluable in learning to diagnose various ailments and that the school would provide an "ample" supply of patients to complete their clinical requirements. Similar representations were made in literature used to recruit them.

- Implicit in these representations was a promise that the students would not only earn a chiropractic degree but would acquire sufficient skills in the diagnosis and treatment of physical ailments to enable passage of their home state licensing examinations.

- When the students approached their final year and eligibility to work in the Clinic as student interns, the school's faculty told them that, to meet the minimum clinical experience required for graduation, they would have to recruit patients from among their friends, family members, neighbors, co-workers, and, in some cases, complete strangers.

- Although the Clinic director told one student that the school had never promised to provide patients, some student overheard admission representatives making the very same representations to prospective students touring the clinic.

- Although some students had patients "passed down" to them by graduating interns, many students who received no "pass-down" patients and were not from Kansas city were unable to recruit enough patients to graduate on time. School representative encouraged these students to "market themselves" in the community and create their own "mini-practice" by using the school's spinal screening equipment to interest patients in the Clinic. One student who found that this was not enough was advised by a faculty member to "cold-call" prospective patients listed in the Kansas City telephone directory.

- While solicitation and marketing efforts enabled students to eventually meet the *quantitative* requirements for clinical service, they were not able to develop the diagnostic skills necessary for chiropractic practice because most of the recruited individuals were generally symptom-free and did not need any major chiropractic adjustment.

- Adding insult to injury, the school profited handsomely or had the fees paid by the patients or by the students themselves on the patients' behalf for any treatments (whether needed or not) that the patients received.

- As a result of inadequate instruction, the plaintiffs were not adequately prepared to pass their board examinations and were unable to enter into a chiropractic practice due to lack of basic experience in diagnosis. Virtually all of the plaintiffs found it necessary to take review and preparatory courses (at additional cost) before sitting for their respective board examinations. Some felt that their practical experience was so lacking that they were forced to educate themselves as unpaid interns under the tutelage of licensed chiropractors in their home states. This deficiency was a direct result of the school's failure to provide an "ample volume and variety of patients" to allow the students to relate their classroom education to real-world patients who had acute ailments and symptoms.

Not the First Lawsuit

In a 1996 lawsuit, the jury awarded $93,000 in actual damages plus $45,000 in punitive damages to Julie Bernet, a former CCC student. She stated that to meet quotas, students were required to lure friends and family into the schools clinic and then charge them for chiropractic treatment they did not need [4]. At the trial, a former instructor testified that, between 1991 and 1995, she knew of no student who met the clinical requirements solely by relying on patients provided by the clinic [5]. The case was later settled for an undisclosed sum [1]. Her affidavit in the case follows.

Lawsuit References

1. Trokyna et al v. Cleveland Chiropractic College, Civil action No. 99-0746-CV-W-2. Filed Aug 3, 1999, in the United States District Court for the Western District of Missouri.
2. Morris M. Chiropractic College students file suit. Class says recruiting patients was a part of the requirements. *Kansas City Star*, Aug 5, 1999, pB2.
3. Jury finds for former chiropractic students on one point, school on two. *Associated Press*, Nov 29, 2000.
4. Burnet J. Affidavit, April 12, 1996.
5. Menninger B. Student policies questions in school verdict. *Kansas City Business Journal*, July 12-18, 1996, pp. 1,42.

Julie Bernet Affidavit

This affidavit was filed on April 12, 1996 during Julie Bernet's suit against Cleveland Chiropractic College.

State of Missouri

County of Jackson

1. At the time I was being recruited by Cleveland Chiropractic College to enroll as a student, I based my decision to enroll upon my belief that the representations made to me by the admissions representative were true. Additionally, I relied upon the truth of the statements in CCC's printed brochures, handbooks and other literature.

2. While visiting the college for the first time in 1990, I was advised by the CCC admissions representative that my clinical experience would

involve treating sick and injured public patients who sought out chiropractic treatment at the clinic. The admissions representative seriously misrepresented the nature of the clinical experience. Contrary to her assurances that I would fulfill my clinical requirements with patients provided to me by the clinic, I learned at the beginning of the seventh trimester that in fact I would have to round up friends and acquaintances so I could experiment on them and practice chiropractic manipulation. By this time I had already invested an enormous amount of time and money in this education and felt I was forced to remain. Had the admissions counselor been honest with me during the admission process and admitted that the clinic was merely a money making venture for the college, designed to force the students to drag in their friends and family and charge them for unnecessary manipulation, I would have never enrolled at this disreputable institution.

3. In particular, I was assured that when it came time for me to complete the clinical portion of my studies that I would be provided with an ample volume and variety of patients by CCC. The admissions representative stressed that my clinical experience at CCC would involve treating real patients that came to the clinic with genuine physical problems including a wide variety of pathologies which would allow me to gain a diverse experience in the clinical setting. This was absolutely untrue. Once I had entered the clinic I found that the school rarely attracted legitimate patients with genuine physical problems that required the types of chiropractic treatments necessary for successful completion of my clinical requirements. The clinic was described to me as just that, a clinic where sick patients came for chiropractic treatment. It was never explained to me by the admissions I personnel that the clinic was a money-making venture for Cleveland Chiropractic College and that the student was required to lure or entice friends and family into the clinic, and then charge them for chiropractic treatment which they did not need.

4. Contrary to the oral assurances of the admissions personnel and the written representations made in the college's brochures such as deposition Exhibit 8 attached hereto as Exhibit 1, the Cleveland Chiropractic Clinic never provided an ample volume and variety of patients to the students. Rather, the vast majority of "patients" were really not patients at all. We were urged by the clinic director...to recruit any and everyone we knew into the clinic to practice chiropractic upon them, whether they needed it or not. At the suggestion of my supervising clinicians, most of my "patients" were, in reality, friends and family who

I wanted to assist me in obtaining the necessary requirements for the clinic so I could graduate.

5. During my second visit to CCC but prior to my decision to enroll, I visited the CCC with my parents. During that visit we met with an admissions representative or counselor of CCC. My father is a college administrator and asked very specific questions about how I would fulfill the clinical requirements. The admissions representative made it perfectly clear that my clinical requirements would be satisfied by treating patients that the clinic provided me from the general public who came to the clinic with legitimate physical problems. My experience in the clinic proved these statements to be absolutely untrue. Sometime during trimester seven, I was advised for the first time that it would be my responsibility to lure my friends and family in so I could manipulate their necks and backs. The vast majority of the chiropractic treatment rendered in the clinic was being performed on the students' friends and families, as myself and other students desperately sought volunteers that we could work on.

6. At the conclusion of the second meeting with the college's admissions personnel I was given a tour of the clinic itself. My parents accompanied us on this tour which was conducted by the admissions personnel attempting to persuade me to enroll. At the time of the tour I was very curious as to the types of patients I would be treating in the clinic. The admissions representative assured me and said that I would be exposed to a wide range of patients who either walked in from the street or were referred into the clinic for public chiropractic treatment. I was repeatedly assured that the school would be responsible for recruiting and procuring a sufficient volume and variety of chiropractic patients for me to complete my training and education.

7. I was also told during my tour of the clinic that the waiting room was always full of patients waiting for the student clinicians to treat. Once I had reached the point in my education where I was involved in the clinic I found this to be completely untruthful.

8. One of the most basic functions a chiropractor performs on each patient is the taking of a physical. A physical involves conducting a detailed examination of the patient to assess the individual's need, if any, for chiropractic treatment. In order to satisfy that portion of my clinical experience dealing with physicals, I was required to complete 20 physicals. Although the admissions representative represented that the

school would provide these patients, I recruited 13 or 14 of the 20 patients that I did physicals on.

9. Because I did not know a large number of people in the Kansas City area with serious neck and back problems, I was frequently forced to recruit patients for treatment who did not have any serious neck or back problems. Once my friends arrived at the clinic I was always given the approval of the supervising clinicians to perform spinal adjustments. I frequently was allowed to adjust friends and acquaintances necks and backs who were, at the time, experiencing no neck or back pain or problems. Deposition Exhibit 8 stated that "students are taught how to care about patients as well as how to care for them" which was not true. The focus of my clinical experience was that the staff clinicians constantly stressed the need for me to recruit patients off the street, namely, my friends and acquaintances. An inordinate amount of time and energy was focused on teaching me how to generate income for the clinic by recruiting friends and acquaintances into the clinic for treatment that they would not otherwise have needed or sought treatment for....

10. I first became aware that I had been lied to concerning the clinical portion of the program shortly following my starting the student intern program. This was in the seventh trimester in school. This was the beginning of my last year of education or my third year.

11. The hearing committee was not comprised of neutral parties because Dr. Moore had already decided to find against me.

12. The due process committee would not allow me to have counsel present.

13. I was not allowed to attend the hearing and, in fact, I was not permitted to confront or question any witnesses. I did not even know who the witnesses were against me. I was forced to remain seated in the hallway while my expulsion hearing was going on.

14. I neither falsified nor altered records, but merely reduced the charge made by the clinic to a patient that I was forced to repeatedly drag into the clinic in order to satisfy my clinical requirements. This was a common practice at the clinic for students to reduce charges on patients they were forced to drag into the clinic for unnecessary adjustments, which the college not only condoned, but encouraged, in order to generate revenue for the clinic.

15. After the expulsion, the financial burden that I was left with, my lack of prospects for redeeming my career as a chiropractor and the time I had spent training and the humiliation prompted me to attempt suicide.

16. At the time I was expelled, I had completed all of my requirements for graduation with the exception of a few clinical requirements.

17. At the time of my enrollment, I was shown a promotional brochure identical to the "View Book", which is marked as Exhibit 1.

18. I agreed to the rules and regulations policies and procedures in the 1991-1992 School Catalog. I was never even given a 1994 or 1995 catalog and certainly received no consideration for any rules changes made by Cleveland. Nor have I agreed to abide by rules and regulations drafted years after my enrollment.

19. I did not transfer to another chiropractic college because of my disenchantment and disgust with chiropractic. Contrary to the representations made by the admissions representative, I have learned through their clinic that CCC encourages unnecessary chiropractic manipulation. Had I have known that true nature of operation of a chiropractic clinic I would have never enrolled.

I, Julie Bernet, first being duly sworn on my oath states that the above statements are true to the best of my knowledge and belief.

~ ~ ~ ~ ~

Essentially, when I was in college and years later, if you were a student and wanted to graduate you had to supply most if not all of your own patients. Stories circulated that some students hired prostitutes to do breast exams on and do blood draws on to fulfill clinic requirements for graduation.

School's Out, Self-Employed and On My Own

Where would I launch my own practice? I had decided on Mesa, Arizona. I wanted to return to the Phoenix area, having spent two years there in high school, and eager to get to a warm climate where I could play golf. I picked Mesa because it was in the path of growth for the metro Phoenix area. I got a map and put colored pins in it, one for each chiropractor, osteopath or GP. Then I picked a pin-free zone on the map and rented office space in a strip mall there.

My wife helped me get the office ready and plan a ribbon-cutting ceremony. I invited everyone I knew and many I did not, including the mayor. Twelve people showed up. Twelve friends and relatives, zero patients. Zero mayors.

I got my first patient thanks to my wife. She walked door-to-door in the neighborhoods behind the clinic, introducing the clinic and handing out cards. One of those cards brought in a middle-aged woman with back problems, a school cafeteria lady who stood all day. I had my first real patient. I taught her exercises, and did three or four adjustments over the next weeks. Her back got better, and although I have not seen her in a decade, she still sends me referrals.

My goal for my practice was simple: make it through five years. I had read the statistics that ninety percent of businesses fail in the first five years, so I assumed that if I made it to five, the rest would follow. Those five years were some of the most wretched of my life. The patients did not materialize the way I had assumed they would. My income was less than my overhead. At one point I had to choose between my utility bills and my college loan payments.

I visited with two consultants who promised to teach me the secrets of success. I learned in a "practice building seminar" that the successful chiropractor sees each patient an average of thirty or more times. One doctor who was held up to us as a hero, a star, managed to see his patients an average of 56 times.

My own average was woeful -- perhaps three visits. I gave most patients exercises, then told them to return if they did not get better. So the economics were simple enough. In today's dollars a chiropractic visit might cost $40. It is usually less than $30 if it is Medicare or Workers' Comp, and as high as $120 if it is an insurance case, such as an auto accident. But, for a typical bad back case, the fee is, say, $40. I was seeing a person three times, for a total of $120. The guy who averaged 56 times could expect to get $2,240 from the same patient.

The consultants taught us to increase the average visits by following a step-by-step list, one that advised you to tell every patient, "You have a serious problem." Then, after letting that bit of bad news settle in, you were to tell them they needed several visits before being re-evaluated. If they did not improve over the course of those visits, well, then, they needed more frequent visits. If they got better, you warned them to keep coming if they wanted to avoid relapses.

Following the practice-building sessions, the first new patient I saw was a young woman experiencing mid-back pain. My examination revealed that she had had an injury years before, long enough for arthritis to have fused two vertebrae together. She was young for this, but then she had been a competitive gymnast and had probably suffered an injury during her athletic career.

Once the vertebrae are fused, adjustments will not help. All she could do was strengthen the surrounding muscles. Adhering to an exercise regimen, she could function normally.

As I sat down with her and her parents to review my diagnosis, I knew there was not much I could do to help her, besides the exercises. Still, my new marketing training told me what to do: tell her she had a serious problem. Scare her. Then give her a long series of adjustments.

I sat with her, my step-by-step marketing list discreetly inside a folder so I could follow my script and recruit her as a regular. But as I looked down on this sweet, tiny ex-gymnast, **I just could not do it.** I could not give her a scare that would haunt her, perhaps for life, limiting her activities, maybe even affecting decisions such as the one about bearing children. No, instead of scaring her, I tried to inspire her to follow her exercises and surmount her old injury. Then I watched her and her purse walk out the door. Never again did I try to follow the "practice building" script.

Although I was healing backs, I was going broke doing it. Despite believing that I was the best around, I was far from the most visible. The Phoenix area is full of aggressively marketed chiropractors that could afford things like full-page ads in the Yellow Pages. All of them followed the same basic marketing plan: offer free services. Free x-rays or free examination. It reminded me of those early anti-drug films they showed us in high school: "the first one is always free." But the first one was free because there were thirty or more to come. For me, it was one free of two or three or four. I believed that I was offering superior services, but it was the other chiropractors that could afford to run the ads and offer the freebies.

My solution was to conduct seminars. I offered myself as a speaker, explaining my view of chiropractic healing. Little did I know that my career, and my life, was about to change forever.

Chapter 3

My Change of Life

I tried to make money as a kid. I had a lemonade stand for about six weeks. I made no money. I had to burn it down and collect insurance.

~ **Brian Kiley**

One of my first speaking engagements was for an audience of 400 insurance adjusters and attorneys. I was one of three speakers. An orthopedic surgeon and a physical therapist were the other two. The surgeon was arrogant and obtuse, slouching over the lectern and shooting from the expensively-tailored hip. The therapist was likable, but likewise unprepared, merely ad-libbing. In contrast, I came with thirty pages of handouts, copies for everyone in the crowd. I delivered a carefully rehearsed speech. Afterwards, I was practically mobbed. Everyone wanted my business card and my opinion. They asked if I did peer reviews and IMEs. Even though I had been in business for five years, I had never heard of either one. Later I learned that an IME is an Independent Medical Examination ~ a second opinion following an examination of the patient. A peer review is also a second opinion, but without the patient exam, just a review of a doctor's records. This was the beginning of my work as an expert witness, and the beginning of my being hated by many local chiropractors.

In the late 1980s, I was asked by a nurse-consulting group to speak at a seminar on how to treat whiplash. In the audience of some 400 people were plaintiff lawyers, insurance adjusters, and defense lawyers. I talked about how I had been seeing a change in the literature, suggesting that less treatment is probably better for whiplash patients ~ the victims of rear end car accidents. I advocated that home care ~ including exercise ~ should be emphasized over passive treatments such as ice and heat massage.

Whiplash was and unfortunately still can be the golden goose for chiropractors. This is because the practitioners were rarely challenged on the $5,000-per patient bills they routinely submitted to insurance companies for providing whiplash treatment. My seminar audience -- who dealt frequently with chiropractors and their patients-- had never heard a chiropractor suggest that it was better medicine to deliver less treatment, which coincidently keeps costs down. Keeping costs down can be a secondary benefit to providing true evidence-based care.

Afterward, once again someone from the audience asked me to do a "peer review" of another chiropractor's treatment plan for a patient. They also wanted an independent medical exam of the patient. At the time I did not fully understand what those activities were. I simply completed a review of the findings, examined the patient, and submitted my opinion. I did not even realize that I was expected to send a bill for my services! I was not aware I could charge for simply providing a scientific opinion – something my school had conveniently neglected to teach me!

Independent Medical Examinations

The IMEs are typically part of litigation where it is insurance company versus chiropractor and their attorney/client. The case has developed because there is a particularly large bill that the insurance adjuster questions. For instance, one woman was involved in a car accident and her initial chiropractor visit was $3,300. Since that is something like 82 times the cost of a regular office visit, the insurance company was skeptical. The typical scenario goes like this: Someone is injured in an accident. They seek out a chiropractor. The insurance company pays for months of treatment then begin to question the need for additional treatment. At some point they may refuse payment, whereupon the chiropractor – with an attorney might sue. If this develops, that is when the insurance company calls me in to do an IME.

Often the patients are told by their chiropractor or attorney that I am "a company doctor" out to deny them treatment. I am portrayed as such an ogre that some patients come in terrified while others come in belligerent. One man brought a gun. Even though he was in a hospital gown for the examination, he kept his .45 on the examination table throughout. A woman brought a stun gun and held it against her chest the entire time, switching hands as necessary for me to complete the exam.

Sometimes the patients had received excellent care. Sometimes they received *too much* care. I had a patient tell me that her back was just fine after four visits. "Why did you go seventy more times?" I asked.

"My doctor said I should."

Sometimes the patients have simply been misdiagnosed. One woman had been receiving spinal alignments -- the typical "subluxation" -- for a year, 120 visits. That's every three days!. But the real problem was bursitis in her hip. After three sessions of physical therapy she was fine.

✔ Of course, sometimes the doctor is simply inept. Consider this case: A man had low-back problems. His chiropractor's diagnosis was that one of the vertebrae in his neck was out of alignment. So the chiropractor pushed it back, but over-corrected, putting it out of the alignment to the other side. On the following visit, the doctor repeated the error in the other direction. This went on for 202 visits (!) - push left one time, right the next.

✔ Then there are the patients who participate in an insurance scam. Believe me, they know exactly what they are doing. One woman, with remarkable honesty, told me that she was visiting a chiropractor only because she was given up-front money to be a patient – a patient with good insurance.

Few are so honest. In fact, you cannot count on them to even tell the truth about their names. We ended up with so many "examinees" with aliases that I implemented a policy that I would not do the exam unless the examinee could produce photo identification.

Stories That Speak for Themselves!

The most entertaining cases involve the fringes of chiropractic. In this book's Introduction, Dale Dauten spoke of his favorite examples - the man who did the aura adjustments using photographs and x-rays, and the diagnosis of "bruised karma." My own favorites are these:

✔ A chiropractor in Sedona, Arizona, a favorite spot for New Agers, had a large crystal that was rented out to other chiropractors so they can recharge their own, smaller crystals.

✔ A chiropractor who consults with a colleague on some of his patients, which would not be remarkable except the colleague in question has been dead for 400 years. The chiropractor gets the opinions by channeling a 15th century Scottish physician.

I find such stories amusing, but there are too many that are alarming, revealing the dark side of the profession:

✔ A male chiropractor who would insert his thumb in a woman's vagina and his index finger in her anus. His purpose, he claimed, was to "balance her harmonics."

✔ Another chiropractor did rectal exams on all his female patients. Chiropractors, generally, are not allowed to practice internal medicine. That was bad enough, but he also videotaped each rectal exam. His explanation? That if his bills were questioned, he wanted proof that he had in fact performed this procedure. This is an unnecessary and, in most places, illegal procedure.

✔ There was also a chiropractor who was treating cancer with an orange light. It was just an orange light bulb in a wooden box.

After a decade of doing IME and peer reviews, and testifying in legal proceedings, I have come to see the worst in chiropractic medicine. Without intending to, I have become an expert in scams and ineptitude. I wish I could say that it is rare, a tiny percentage, but over the years I have come to believe that thanks to mistreatment and especially to over-treatment, the majority of chiropractic visits are without medical justification.

I have been called many unpleasant names by chiropractors that disagree, but the one label I have chosen to wear with pride is "heretic." Truth is, I did not want to be the expert – it was my telling the truth that made me an expert.

Still, I have not completely left the chiropractic profession. I still treat patients, still fight the good fight against back pain. Nothing gives me more satisfaction than to take patients who have been all but immobilized by back problems, and help them get their lives back.

Psychology pioneer Sigmund Freud once wrote that a man with a toothache cannot fall in love. Well, a man with a backache not only cannot fall in love, but has to struggle to be lovable. A man with a backache cannot play with his children or ride a bike. A woman with a bad back cannot go dancing or rollerblading or hiking. Some cannot even sit through a movie or go to a party. Back pain is robbing millions of people of their joys.

A good, honest chiropractor could help many of those people. Even the old nemesis of chiropractors, the American Medical Association, has stated that chiropractic treatments might be effective. Other studies have concluded that spinal manipulation is the most effective way to treat back injuries. Yet many bad backs belong to people who refuse to even consider chiropractors. Who can blame them?

I decided to write this book because spinal manipulation can be of benefit to a small subset of patients, and because I want to reach out to anyone with back, joint, and muscle pain. They need to know how and where they can find relief.

> ***I want to drive home this very simple and educational fact of life. Acute back pain has a natural history of six weeks. Acute pain is temporary; most lower back injuries are of this type. This means whether you seek treatment or not, you will improve.***

If you are inpatient and seek care, regardless what care you decide upon, your back problems should improve as the natural history of six weeks elapses. In 85-95% of mechanical back pain, strains and sprains, this is an accurate statement. All others might require re-evaluation and additional care, but chances are in your favor that you will not be that special case.

So, your back pain is probably a do it yourself project. What you do before and after an episode of acute back pain for yourself is more important than what any provider might do for you. Passive care is treatment rendered to you, spinal manipulation and heat/cold etc. Active care is what you do for yourself, to strengthen muscles, weight control etc. Throughout this book, always think in terms of what you can do for yourself. Think of how you will heal. Do not think of your back as something you need to go have fixed.

The right mindset can save you time, money, and maybe your life!

Chapter 4

From the Offbeat to the Fraudulent

Everyone is entitled to his own opinion, but not his own facts.

~ Daniel Patrick Moynihan

"You want to do what?" the woman asked incredulously. She was in her early 70s, attractive and fit. She smoothed her dress nervously as she sat in the chiropractor's exam room. She glanced at her husband, whose jaw had slackened.

"Pubic hair analysis," the chiropractor repeated calmly. "It can reveal a lot about your overall health."

The practitioner had met the couple at a community "health fair" and had convinced them to come into his office for a free consultation.

The husband and wife reluctantly agreed. They knew little about chiropractic, but thought it was a reasonable possibility that their occasionally achy backs were causing other medical problems. They were expecting to hear that spinal manipulation might benefit them both.

The chiropractor never performed manipulation on them—at least of the spinal variety. Instead, almost as soon as he entered the exam room, he suggested an eye-popping alternative.

Amazingly, the couple did not bolt out of the office. They submitted to the "analysis" and afterward, were given shocking news. The wife was perhaps hours away from suffering a stroke. She would need a 24-week vitamin therapy regimen at a cost of $33,000.

Out of fear she was dying she went to the Mayo Clinic for testing. All test procedures came back with negative results. She ended up filing a board complaint against her chiropractor.

As disturbing as this story is, it is not an isolated incident. Across the country, more and more consumers are reporting and taking legal action against practitioners of unprofessional, unethical, unproven and medically risky approaches. This coincides with chiropractors having one of the highest satisfaction rates of any health care practitioners among consumers. How can this dichotomy be explained?

Chiropractic is the epitome of "touchy-feely" health care. Typically, as practitioners massage you, they apply pressure to your back and neck—all within the legitimate boundaries of the profession. It can be a soothing, relaxing, reassuring way to spend half an hour or so.

But, when chiropractors suggest or actually perform bogus assessments, recommend therapies they are clearly not qualified to administer, claim to cure life-threatening or chronic conditions or invent treatments and diagnostic tests with no scientific foundation, patients who are naturally skeptical may begin to question the practitioner's intentions, motivations, skills and experience.

Increasing numbers of chiropractors ignore signs of serious illness in patients as they lead patients to believe that chiropractic is the magic bullet for everything from migraine headaches to cancer.

✔ A Canadian woman who went to a chiropractor for relief of migraine headaches later died from what the coroner determined was a stroke brought on by chiropractic adjustment. The woman had complained about the manner in which her neck had been adjusted and the intense pain that followed her treatment. By the way, migraines start in the brain, not the spinal column.

✔ A school bus driver stepped off the bus, slipped on a patch of ice and fell, hitting the middle of his back on the bus steps. After driving himself to the local chiropractor, he began conventional treatment. The chiropractor never performed an exam and did not order x-rays. One day, after two months of regular chiropractic adjustments, the patient was unable to get out of bed. He was taken to a hospital where x-rays revealed he had three compression fractures in his thoracic spine~ the middle part of the back ~ and cancer. Just months later, he died.

✔ A man in Missouri diagnosed with AIDS was experiencing back pain and sought treatment from a chiropractor. Ultimately, the chiropractor convinced the man that he was cured of AIDS and could safely start a family. The patient eventually died of the disease, leaving behind a wife and daughter infected with HIV.

When A Chiropractic Adjustment Is Not What You Need

The public uses the terms "manipulation" and "adjustment" interchangeably, because people not trained in spinal anatomy typically do not understand the difference. Frankly, I did not understand the difference until the early 1990s, and I had been in practice for about eight years at that point. I have learned that the contrast between spinal manipulation and a chiropractic adjustment is profound.

A chiropractic adjustment is based on the premise that a bone in the cervical (upper), thoracic (middle) or lumbar (lower) spine is out of place and must be put back into proper alignment. Chiropractors call these out-of-place bones "subluxations" and claim that they cause nerve pressure that leads to disease. No one has ever been able to prove that subluxations exist. And, if you think about it logically, how could you function at all--how could you not be experiencing paralysis---if a spinal bone is out of alignment? If you were to view an x-ray of a patient with an actual "C-5" fracture - a fracture of the fifth vertebra of the cervical spine - you would very likely be looking at a paralyzed patient. A chiropractor is attempting—through an adjustment—to restore the identified "out-of-place" bone to its rightful place in your spinal column. He or she probably will tell you that it took many years to knock that bone out of alignment and it may take a very long time - perhaps as many as forty-two visits! - to fully correct the "subluxation." After the subluxation is finally corrected, you will then be told that additional visits are needed to "stabilize" you.

A spinal manipulation, on the other hand, has been shown from evidence-based medicine to be the most effective treatment of choice for acute back pain. Spinal manipulation involves applying pressure on the back in the area that is no longer functioning as optimally as it has in the past and where movement has become restricted as a result of strain, overuse, poor posture or age. The region's decrease in function is what causes back pain, and the goal of a spinal manipulation is to restore function, increase mobility, and minimize pain. The goal of a spinal manipulation is to loosen up the area by applying appropriate pressure to that region of the spine. This pressure, applied properly, can release the area from its restriction. You may be free of pain in just one or two visits to a practitioner. Though there cannot be a guarantee that the pain will not return at some point, it certainly is not necessary for a patient to continue with office visits as a preventive measure. There is no scientific evidence that continuing chiropractic treatment has any therapeutic benefit.

Spinal manipulation can be empirically proven to help acute back pain. However, chiropractic adjustments cannot be scientifically validated. So why don't chiropractors just focus on spinal manipulations? Because they are not lucrative enough. Many chiropractors have figured out that it makes much more sense to concentrate on correcting subluxations, because they can insist that it will take thirty visits or so to realize success.

The irony is that chiropractors probably would ultimately treat 100 percent of the population that complains of back pain – about eighty percent of all Americans – if they restricted their practices to evidence-based spinal manipulations. This is in sharp contrast with the ten percent of American who visit chiropractors today.

Instead, chiropractors focus on an approach that has not been proven since 1895 when D.D. Palmer introduced his theory of chiropractic. Chiropractors have become experts at quoting legitimate studies about the benefits of spinal manipulation and equating this technique with chiropractic adjustment.

Chiropractors work with a single atom of possibility: there is room to believe that a bone *may* be out of place. They have become the penultimate "spin doctors," expanding that atom of possibility into an entire universe where only they and their patients reside. The entire medical community – with the exception of chiropractic practitioners – does not recognize subluxations or chiropractic adjustments as legitimate – and never will.

Remember this: it is all to make money. But chiropractors can dazzle you with doubt, making you think that if there is even a scintilla of plausibility in their contention, the treatment they offer might be worth a try.

Patients are often told that chiropractic care is the cure for almost any medical problem in any part of the body. Patients or prospective patients are even told that chiropractic can resolve chromosomal anomalies or improve brain function.

✔ A chiropractor told the mother of a speech-delayed two-year-old that a subluxation was the likely culprit for her toddler's limited verbal ability. The chiropractor urged the mother to bring the child to his office for a spinal adjustment. "The speech center is at the base of the brain," the chiropractor said. "If we can bring his spine back into alignment, it may help him speak." For the record, the speech center in the human brain is nowhere near the base of the brain. It is located in the frontal lobe. Good thing for this patient the doc was a chiropractor and not a brain surgeon.

✔ A chiropractor told the mother of a Down syndrome baby that he could "cure" the child's condition. The truth? Down syndrome is caused by a genetic aberration of Chromosome 21. Chromosomal abnormalities can never be "cured."

Pediatric Chiropractic Care Lures More Believers

✔ A five-year-old boy and his four-year-old sister both suffered from ear infections but were treated with spinal manipulation instead of antibiotic therapy. Their infections worsened and deteriorated into mastoiditis, an inflammation of the lining of the small cells in the mastoid bone behind the ear. This condition has been extremely rare since antibiotics were introduced after World War II to treat bacterial infections. The little girl lost her hearing in one ear as a result of the mastoiditis.

Incidents like this have been on the rise in the past 25 years as chiropractors expand their practices to welcome newborns, infants, toddlers and older children. Numerous web sites have sprung up simultaneously with chiropractors claiming that childhood diseases and common medical conditions can be prevented and often treated by spinal adjustment. A few web sites that are particularly troubling are those of the International Chiropractic Pediatric Association at **www.4icpa.org**, the International Chiropractic Online Network at **www.chiropage.com/Chiropediatrics/default.htm**, and yourspine.com at **http://yourspine.com**. All of these boldly tout the benefits of chiropractic care for children of all ages. "Is chiropractic safe for your child...?" one site asks. "The answer is YES."

Not so fast. Evidence-based practitioners will almost never treat infants and toddlers unless they are working in collaboration with a medical doctor and they will rarely treat children under 13. That is because chiropractic pediatrics is unnecessary and can, in fact, be dangerous. Children's necks and backs are naturally and normally pliant. Adjustments can make them unstable. Because a young child's spine is flexible it is virtually impossible for an infant's or toddler's spine to get out of place. Adjusting infants' soft bones places unnecessary pressure on the individual vertebrae and the connecting ligaments. If a child has a serious condition such as a tumor, then manipulation can induce paralysis.

A chiropractor believes that if a newborn's spine is not adjusted, the baby may be more likely to die of Sudden Infant Death Syndrome. He is so convinced that "traumatic birth" and the resulting "subluxation" can lead to SIDS that he "adjusted" his own just-born son in the delivery room while the umbilical cord was still attached. The proof that his contention is factual, he says, is that his child never died from SIDS.

According to the National Center for Health Statistics, there are about four million babies born each year in the U.S. Up to 7,000 of those babies die of SIDS. As tragic as that figure is, you can see that the statistical likelihood of a baby dying from SIDS is minuscule. By this chiropractor's logic, every newborn "not adjusted" would be vulnerable to SIDS. That simply is not demonstrated mathematically.

Marvin Levant, M.D., a Canadian physician notes, "With chiropractic, the spinal column is the entryway into a philosophical belief system that the spinal cord is somehow the master of the human body. Every first year medical student knows [that] the notion that the spinal column...somehow controls all our body functions, is an anatomical impossibility. It has never been true and can never be true."

It is virtually if not physically impossible for catastrophic conditions such as SIDS or for asthma, colic, rashes, croup and other common childhood ailments to be linked to the improper alignment of the spine.

Serious bacterial infections frequently require antibiotics. Chiropractors often disparage the use of any drugs, particularly in children. When a chiropractor convinces a parent that a child's middle ear infection can be treated with adjustments only, the parent is being misled and the child is receiving inappropriate care with potentially *devastating complications.*

Chiropractors often belittle not only prescription medications but childhood immunizations as well. They will use scare tactics, warning of the potentially deadly consequences of vaccinations and of "injecting noxious substances into your perfectly healthy child." Their arguments are compelling enough to make even parents who completely trust their M.D.s question the need for immunizations. But remember what Dr. Levant points out: "Chiropractic philosophy maintains the removal of phantom spinal subluxations is the 'natural way' to prevent polio, tetanus, diphtheria, measles, etc." Even if subluxations could be demonstrated, it makes no sense to think that they have any connection whatsoever to systemic infections. **Immunizations — even though they carry some risk — are the best way to protect your child from debilitating childhood diseases.**

Pediatric Chiropractic On The Rise

Actually, this fourth category of chiropractic patients is growing. More and more parents are arranging for a chiropractor to be their children's primary health care provider, buying into the arguments from the chiropractic community that chiropractors are completely qualified to deliver drug-free care for all manner of children's ailments, from ear infections to asthma.

Those arguments are bolstered by the International Chiropractors Association's program that allows one to become a diplomat in pediatric chiropractic. You are required to complete a three-year postgraduate series of courses to be named a diplomat. Sounds fairly rigorous, right? Let us compare it to the hours of residency training required of a recent medical school graduate who wants to be a pediatrician.

The chiropractic three-year program consists of 360 hours and 30 modules or courses. You can complete the coursework on 30 separate weekends over a three-year period. How much do you think they are going to remember from weekend to weekend over a period of 36 months? Pediatricians in training, on the other hand, undergo about 360 hours a month of continual hands-on instruction. They have multiple opportunities every day to care for children with a range of health problems and they maintain nearly constant interaction with experienced pediatricians, pediatric surgeons and other specialists. Medical doctors who are working to become pediatricians have dedicated their adult lives to treating children. Chiropractors who want to become diplomats in pediatrics simply want to expand their patient base. They become diplomats by attending weekend seminars where they sip cocktails in a banquet room and never lay eyes on or examine a pediatric patient except through photographs or videos. Actual pediatricians in training spend days on end for three years or more learning in a hospital environment, trying to bring down a child's extremely high fever or control symptoms of asthma and assisting in surgery, in addition to performing hundreds of other medical tests and procedures for actual patients.

So, honestly, to whom would you rather bring your child? To someone who believes (there is that word again: "believe") that curing middle-ear infections is as easy as a chiropractic adjustment of the neck, or to someone who has had advanced training and has successfully treated hundreds of ear infections based on peer-reviewed clinical protocols? When you bring your child to a chiropractor, not only are you engaging in a risky practice, you are wasting your money, your time and your energy.

Canada takes a much stronger task with chiropractors than the United States. The Pediatric Section of the Alberta Medical Association had the following to say: "Chiropractic use of x-rays of infants and children to diagnose so-called vertebral subluxations is unscientific and of no value whatsoever. Parents should never allow their children's spines to be x-rayed by a chiropractor." The position paper continued," Chiropractic spinal adjustments is NOT required as preventive therapy to maintain a child's health."

The Pediatric Section was not done yet. "There is no scientific evidence whatsoever that the so-called chiropractic spinal adjustments result in any correction of the child's spine. These adjustments are ineffective and useless."

They indicated that no payments be made to chiropractors who treat children under age eighteen, including x-rays. The College of Chiropractors of Alberta were challenged by Canadian Pediatricians to demonstrate subluxations in front of a group of doctors and legislatures; the demonstration never happened.

As one MD put it, "When I contemplate a chiropractor treating a two-week old neonate with a fever, I get a gigantic backache."

It is not just pediatric care that chiropractors routinely claim they are qualified to deliver. Chiropractors frequently expand their practices to include "aura adjustments," nutrition therapy, aromatherapy, homeopathy, acupuncture, "live blood" analysis, cancer treatment and even veterinary chiropractic. The more varied their practice, obviously the more income they can generate.

For the record, "aura adjustments" have no scientific basis. Nutrition therapy, aromatherapy, homeopathy, and acupuncture anecdotally have been shown to have beneficial effects for some patients, but special training is usually required in order for these kinds of approaches to be administered with positive results. Live blood analysis has no medical foundation, and cancer treatment should only be administered by a physician with advanced training in the field of oncology.

Veterinary Chiropractic

Stop for a moment -- just visualize spinal manipulation for dogs, cats, and horses. Unbelievable, isn't it?

Veterinary chiropractic is not legitimate, but it is out there. The chance of injuring a helpless animal – an animal that cannot speak for itself – did not stop one chiropractor from secretly using it on at least one pet of an unsuspecting owner.

✔ The neighbor of a chiropractor was in an automobile accident along with his dog. When he heard that the neighbor and his dog had been in the car wreck, the chiropractor suggested that they both undergo chiropractic adjustments.

The neighbor declined, but the chiropractor was so determined to demonstrate the value of his profession that he climbed over the fence every day for a couple of weeks and secretly adjusted the dog. The dog got better and the chiropractor then revealed to the neighbor what he had done.

The reality is that in eight out of ten cases - be they human, canine or even feline - back pain resolves without any medical intervention. Animals are similar to children in that they cannot communicate effectively or at all concerning their pain thresholds. What easy targets for the less than honest practitioner. Should we call this "Taking advantage of the weak, young, and four-legged?"

Unbelievable, yet weekend seminars are offered in animal chiropractic. Some practitioners devout an entire day to seeing only our furry friends. I guess the possible mistake on the carpet makes it so! There are now "Natural Pet Care Expos" that well-meaning but gullible consumers and their loyal, helpless pets can attend. The interested pet owner can find out how to cure their pet's constipation, be it manipulation to coffee enemas to counseling sessions with a pet therapist. Go figure!

Says David W. Ramey, D.V.M., "No part of chiropractic education deals with animals, and no part of veterinary education deals with manipulative forms of physiotherapy. In most states, the practice of chiropractic is, by definition, restricted to humans." So, what is the reason for the increase in animal chiropractic, you ask. Let us look at the data.

Nearly every one of the 281 million people living in the United States will see a medical doctor or osteopathic physician at least once in their lives. But it is estimated that only ten percent of the total population--about 28 million people--will visit a chiropractor. When you consider that there are approximately 70,000 chiropractors across the United States competing for a relatively limited population of patients, you begin to see why chiropractors market themselves so aggressively. They are, of course, trying to convince even a minute fraction of the remaining 245 million Americans that chiropractic care can dramatically improve the quality of their lives, and mess with their innocent children and animals. Can you say child abuse?

State Board of Chiropractic Examiners

I urge you -- before you go to a chiropractor -- to attend a meeting of your local board of chiropractic examiners, where public complaints about chiropractic care are heard. At that meeting, you are likely to learn about full-body x-rays given to children , exposing them unnecessarily to too much radiation, or highly inappropriate and unprofessional conduct, such as vaginal massage or breast stimulation.

✔ In Pulaski, Virginia a chiropractor told a female patient he could relieve her constipation by massaging her vagina!

✔ Another chiropractor proceeded to perform a breast examination on a female patient by sucking on her right breast. After the patient left his office and called the police, the chiropractor abandoned his practice and, according to police, fled the state.

✔ Yet another chiropractor massaged a woman's breasts, telling her it would decrease her rib inflammation.

✔ Still another treated patients by encouraging them to ride bareback on a horse in a circular motion.

Why Won't Your State Board of Chiropractic Protect You?

You will learn that these boards, typically composed of practicing chiropractors appointed by the state, are infuriatingly reluctant to censure, discipline, or take drastic action against those in their own profession. This board is a buffer to protect their duly licensed chiropractors. You may hear stories of patients who suffered a stroke after a chiropractic adjustment, but you may or may not witness any action against their chiropractors. Though solid data is rare, often suppressed, stroke can be a complication of chiropractic adjustment.

The boards often do not address complaints about excessive fees or excessive treatments. So, although you may hear stories about thousands of dollars spent on dozens of chiropractic visits, do not be surprised if the board replies that it does not consider these types of grievances.

> ***Although you will not witness much action at these meetings, you will hear a litany of complaints that will make you think twice about seeking the services of a chiropractor you know nothing or little about.***

Since the mid-1990s, as I continued to conduct peer reviews and IMEs, I have been exposed to the worst the chiropractic profession has to offer. Here are the most outrageously fraudulent examples of treatment and billing that I have come across:

- Charges of $65,000 from one chiropractor treating one patient
- One patient treated by the same chiropractor for the same condition for ten years
- One patient involved in one auto accident saw a chiropractor 1,200 times
- A patient was billed $3,300 bill for her initial visit to a chiropractor.

When Is A Doctor Not A Doctor?

Chiropractors are allowed to call themselves "doctors". One wonders what medical doctors feel about that. Even though they have not met stringent entrance requirements to obtain their schooling, nor having to prove their techniques and abilities, a chiropractor can call himself a doctor anytime. What "doctor" has completed few prerequisite college courses, has no training directly with patients other than their fellow students, friends and family members, and only had to undertaken an internship that consists almost entirely of watching videos and practicing medicine on models? What "doctor" has learned non-scientific notions instead of medical and anatomical realities?

Be wary of chiropractors that over-emphasize the "doctor" in their title. It may be an attempt to disguise their inadequacies as health care practitioners or artificially enhance their credibility. After all, only 42 percent of chiropractors have earned a bachelor's degrees. Among medical doctors, 99.8 percent have earned undergraduate degrees.

Sucking In Patients

Let us imagine that you are a new chiropractor. You have no patients, but you need some. What do you do?

It is not uncommon for chiropractors to "recruit" patients through accident reports filed with local police departments. Accident reports, which list all auto accidents that occurred the day before, are public record. In one state not long ago, there were so many chiropractors and lawyers requesting reports each day that the local police department began charging $5 for every copy requested. Eventually, when that did not deter them, the department stopped providing copies of accident reports. Some states have passed laws making it illegal to solicit victims of an accident. If soliciting an accident victim were a felony, conviction would bring automatic revocation of a chiropractor's license. Most laws identify such an action as a misdemeanor.

Fishing for patients through police departments or other public agencies can be the tip of the iceberg when it comes to unethical and illegal practices, particularly with regard to filing lawsuits. In many states, the following scenario is illegal, but it still happens far too often. An auto accident occurs. The driver and passengers are approached by someone who says, "If you are looking for a doctor, I would be happy to take you to one right now." This "someone" is known among fraud investigators as a "capper" or a "runner." The doctor conducts an examination and determines that the patient is injured. The capper/runner then volunteers to take the patient immediately to a lawyer's office, and all the parties ~ except the patient in some situations ~ ultimately share in any award that is later received from a lawsuit or settlement.

Today, chiropractic services are covered to some extent by Medicare, Medicaid, workers' compensation and many health insurance plans. President Bush just signed into law chiropractic services at Veterans hospitals/clinics. In one state recently, the state legislature passed a bill that mandates every health maintenance organization to pay for a minimum of twelve chiropractic visits per member, if the member wants chiropractic care. At least 44 other states require at least some insurance coverage of chiropractic care.

Perpetuating Fraud

Some view the government-sanctioned mandatory insurance coverage as an accomplishment for the chiropractic industry. But did you know, insurance is also an excellent opportunity for fraud. Fraud can take the form of fake claims, double charges for patients, and bills for multiple visits when a patient may have only been seen once. The National Crime Insurance Bureau estimates that all fraudulent schemes ~ not just those perpetrated by chiropractors ~cost consumers $20 billion a year. We all bear that burden through higher taxes, higher insurance rates, and ballooning health care costs.

✔ The chiropractor's representative stepped gingerly over the broken glass, rocks, beer bottles, discarded toys, and smelly trash surrounding the housing project in Gary, Indiana. He stopped at one front door, hesitated, then knocked quietly. A young woman answered, two children under four clinging to her threadbare slacks.

"Good afternoon, ma'am," the chiropractor's surrogate began. "I represent a doctor of chiropractic and I want to offer you a chance to give your kids here a chance for first-rate medical care at no cost to you. Our office does not use drugs or give your kids shots or anything like that. We simply examine their spines to make sure their bones are lined up properly. The kids will feel like they are getting a massage."

The woman looked interested, so the visitor continued. "We promise no pain and no risk to your kids and absolutely no cost to you." He handed her a business card and she noticed that the office was located just a couple of miles from her apartment.

"How would I get my kids to this office?" she asked. "I don't have a car."

"That is the great thing," the visitor said, smiling broadly. "We will bring a bus over to your place to pick 'em up. You are welcome to come too. All we need for you to do is sign this permission-to-treat form and provide your Medicaid ID number. We will do the rest."

The woman complied. The weekly treatments for her children consisted of a two-to-five-minute visit that included the use of a temperature gradient study machine. This is a device that records heat and stress along the spine and has never been scientifically proven, but costs hundreds of dollars per treatment.

This story was among dozens uncovered by fraud investigators when they determined that nine of the top ten chiropractors in Gary, Indiana were billing Medicaid operated clinics in three of the poorest counties in the state and had raked in $3.3 million just from those clinics. That amount represented about half of the total amount Medicaid paid to chiropractors statewide.

You might think it is unlikely that you would be approached out of the blue by a chiropractor. Remember the older couple that met the chiropractor at a health fair? Chiropractors' representatives often make unsolicited telephone calls or send direct-mail advertising right to your mailbox. Open it – it is an invitation for free spinal exams for you, your family, children, and maybe even your pets.

The National Insurance Crime Bureau, an agency that works closely with insurance companies and law enforcement agencies who crack down on insurance criminals, warns against unwanted solicitation. Be cautious of anyone who immediately solicits your business following an accident, the agency says. This is easier said than done considering the accident trauma and the pain.

Attention All Auto Accident Victims

✔ If you are ever in an automobile accident and you consult an attorney, be suspicious of a request to see a specific doctor or chiropractor. Attorneys involved in "medical mills" will often insist that accident victims seek medical treatment from a specific health care practitioner.

✔ If you do seek chiropractic care after an accident and the chiropractor recommends multiple visits for minor injuries, seek a second opinion.

✔ Report suspicious activity. If you suspect a provider of health or legal services is using you to falsify an insurance claim, notify the National Insurance Crime Bureau through its toll-free hotline, 1-800-TEL-NICB.

The United States is diligent in its efforts to combat quackery and fraud, but Canada is even more vigilant in protecting the best interests of consumers because the medical community there is especially active in challenging chiropractic dogma. Chiropractic has achieved greater legitimacy in the minds of the populace there than in the U.S. Under Canada's medical system, anyone can visit a chiropractor and have that service paid for by the government. For more about how both the U.S. and Canada are vigorously fighting medical quackery, visit three information-rich consumer advocacy web sites: www.chirowatch.com, www.chirobase.org and www.quackwatch.com.

> ***Fully one-third of healthcare provider fraud is from billing for services never rendered. A chiropractor sees a patient one time and bills for twelve visits is not uncommon in fraud cases. It has been estimated that insurance fraud costs us $30 billion each year. To you that means $200-300 more each year in insurance premium payments.***

To combat fraud of this nature the FBI in 1997 alone received $46 million. In 1998, the FBI had nine squads dedicated to chiropractic fraud at work throughout the United States. Total enforcement activities saw $1.2 billion awarded from negotiations, fines, settlements, and judgments.

More Actual Fraud Cases

It is time to sit back for story hour, just like when you were in grade school. I have compiled a group of fraud cases for you, all true, so enjoy!

✔ In Phoenix, Arizona, ten people were indicted for collecting $350,000.00 in false insurance claims. Two attorneys and a chiropractor staged auto accidents. They went as far as to buy the insurance and "buy" people to cause the accidents. They billed the insurance companies for chiropractic care that was never performed. Once apprehended and brought to justice, one attorney received eight years for his crime.

✔ In Greeneville, South Carolina, a chiropractor defrauded the insurance industry out of $2,000,000 by doing unnecessary nerve and vascular tests. FBI got this one. Good job guys.

✔ In New Jersey, the FBI caught a chiropractor billing for services when the patients were not in town. The chiropractor created false notes in an attempt to protect himself. Didn't work. Another New Jersey case involved fifteen counts of mail fraud. Maximum sentence is five years in federal prison, $250,000 fine, and a continuing relationship with your cellmate named "Killer."

✔ In New York state, a chiropractor was charged in running a $10 million scheme disguising services as medical rehabilitation and false claims.

✔ In Texas, a chiropractor submitted approximately $5.7 million in false claims. This one will serve 2-60 months and pay $2.75 million in restitution.

✔ From Missouri, here is a case worth repeating: a chiropractor had his license suspended for convincing a Mennonite Farmer with AIDS that he was cured. The chiropractor went so far as telling the farmer to have a family. The farmer died and his wife and daughter, you guessed it, have HIV.

✔ A cocaine-addicted Philadelphia chiropractor pleaded guilty to 54 counts of mail fraud. Being "bi-polar," he was sent to a half-way house and ordered to pay a $15,000 fine. I guess they figured he would have more fun at a half-way house than he would have in jail.

✔ Once again, in New Jersey, two chiropractors were accused of killing their mother and burying her under the driveway. They had already had fraud problems, so one had his license revoked and the other retired.

Not surprising then, with the FBI on the job, from 1992-1999 the U.S. has more than quadrupled the rate of convictions for criminal health fraud. As managed care, evidence-based medicine, and clinical guidelines become more established, you can count on even more fraud stories to appear. But, do not expect your state board of chiropractic examiners to broadcast them.

It is very easy to become so cynical about chiropractic care that the baby is thrown out with the bath water. That is, reputable, appropriate, truly helpful, evidence-based spinal manipulation is shunned because of suspicions about unprofessional and risky behavior among far too many chiropractors. I have no doubt that millions of people will continue to seek help from both ethical and unscrupulous chiropractors.

> ***There can be legitimate benefits from spinal manipulation if it is sought for the correct reasons. You just need to know the right time to visit the practitioner who performs spinal manipulations, because the bottom line is this: proper spinal manipulation can get rid of your back pain, but "chiropractic adjustments" can rip you off and keep you chronically dependent on treatments.***

Chapter 5

Hope For Those In Pain

The best interest of the patient is the only interest to be considered.

~ William J. Mayo

Chiropractors typically enjoy success by relying on the "Placebo Principle." It is an amazingly simple theory: if patients believe they are getting proper care, they frequently start to feel better. If a chiropractor can convince you that the pain in your back is from a "subluxation" instead of a legitimate medical concern and that fifty separate "adjustments" will cure your problem, your outlook may start to improve just from a specious explanation and having your condition diagnosed, however inaccurately. Henry K Beecher, M.D. did a study[4] in 1950 and said the placebo effect was up to 35% of a therapeutic modality. Another study published had the therapeutic benefit of spinal manipulation at 17%. You do the math!

This Placebo Principle approach obviously presents ethical concerns. It detracts from the patient's ability to actively participate in his or her care. The patient does not function independently from the practitioner.

Chiropractors treat essentially healthy people who have short-term back and neck pain. But, to profit more from their practice – pay the bills, etc. – many chiropractors want patients to *believe* their problems can become chronic or can only be cured through more chiropractic care.

All of the stories in the previous chapter and the Placebo Principle notwithstanding, there are some reputable, reliable, evidence-based practitioners who want their patients' medical issues to resolve promptly and completely, and will take whatever appropriate steps are necessary to ensure that each patient gets precisely the attention their medical condition demands.

I will use the term "evidence-based practitioner" in place of "chiropractor" in most cases when talking about a health care professional who provides appropriate, medically justified treatment to

[4] "The Power of the Placebo" JAMA; 1955; 159:1602-1606

patients. "Chiropractor" generally will apply to a more typical practitioner who believes in subluxations and in "chiropractic adjustment" as the cure or preventative measure for a wide range of ills.

When judging remember this: the evidence-based practitioner does not view himself or herself as the pre-eminent authority on a patient's problems. Rather, they are a member of the patient's health care team. In addition to proper chiropractic care, the evidence-based practitioner's approach can run the gamut from candidly telling a patient, "Your problem will resolve on its own" to referring the patient to a medical doctor who specializes in spinal disorders.

Here is an example. For several months Carl Windsor[5] had neck pain that became progressively severe. The pain diminished occasionally, only to recur after a brief respite. He sought help from the chiropractor who was treating his wife. She was having an "adjustment" every week! The chiropractor performed adjustments on Carl for a few weeks then urged him to sign up for a program of sixteen more visits at a cost of $240. Carl decided to think about it.

Shortly afterward, he noticed that his left arm was smaller than his right arm. He could not golf well and his fingers were going numb. Ironically, he and a true evidence-based practitioner met on the golf course.

When the practitioner introduced himself to Carl, he noticed how stiffly Carl held his neck and how his fingers wrapped clumsily around the club as he was teeing off. The practitioner also noticed that Carl was a lousy golfer.

By the ninth hole the practitioner offered to perform spinal manipulation, telling Carl that if he was not significantly better after two or three visits he would be referred to a specialist.

Carl arrived for his first visit. An examination was performed of his cervical and thoracic spine. The diagnosis was classic: he had a ruptured disk in his cervical spine. The best solution was surgery.

"You are a chiropractor and you are recommending surgery?" Carl asked. "Any other chiropractor I have ever been to has talked about surgery as an absolute last resort. They have talked about it being risky and more often than not, unnecessary. Why is surgery the answer for me?"

"Because the problem has not resolved in several months," the practitioner told him. "Chiropractic care will only make you chronically

---

[5] Not his real name.

dependent on treatments that will not cure your problem. I believe surgery that repairs the disk-is what you need." This type of surgery is a very straightforward, commonly performed procedure.

Carl was referred to a world-renowned neurosurgeon who happened to practice at a prestigious medical facility. The surgeon's diagnosis mirrored the golfing chiropractor's. Carl underwent reparative surgery within two weeks. "The surgery was textbook," Carl later wrote in a letter. "The recovery went well also." Unfortunately, Carl's golf game improved only slightly.

You deserve an honest chance at evidence-based medical care. The following story from an evidence-based practitioner underscores the value of objective decision-making on the part of the practitioner:

"I have had several patients who have been long-time chiropractic patients and have been adjusted two to three times per week for years on end. After I evaluate them, it becomes apparent to me that their problem is hypermobility." Hypermobility is excessive, painful movement. "They lack stability in their muscles and ligaments. When I explain to them that chiropractic adjustments are contra-indicated in their case, they usually become agitated and leave to find another chiropractor who will continue the adjustments on a frequent basis.

"I saw a young female in her late twenties who was complaining of frequent neck pain, intermittent headaches and constant popping in her neck. She had been under chiropractic care for the past two years and had undergone in excess of 200 adjustments. After the evaluation I explained to her that she was hypermobile and that further manipulation was contra-indicated. I wanted her to start on a stabilization exercise program that could be done at home. She was somewhat skeptical and continued to insist on manipulation, which I refused. Instead, I insisted that she give the exercises a try. I spoke with her weekly and after two weeks she began to notice a significant decrease in neck pain and headaches. After four weeks she was asymptomatic.

"Several months later I received a call from a neurosurgeon in North Carolina who wanted to talk about her. Although I was rather concerned, it turned out that he was her father. Her ongoing chiropractic care had been a significant point of contention in the family. The father and I had a very pleasant discussion after that and the daughter continues to see me on a very infrequent basis."

In summary, the patients have surrendered their skepticism due to the sweet song of the chiropractor and do not want to believe that the treatments are not helping them. The patient does not want to admit they made a wrong decision.

It is rare for a chiropractor to turn away patients who insist on spinal manipulation. These are, after all, the patients who epitomize the Placebo Principle and can generate significant revenue for the chiropractor. But among ethical practitioners, manipulations are performed only when there is medical evidence to support such an approach.

> ***How do you know what the medical evidence is? While the real medical evidence may be some rather dry reading, remember this: a professional, compassionate evidence-based chiropractor regards himself or herself as a true "practitioner" who looks to clinical science for guidance and vigorously guards the best interests of the patient initially, along the way, and ultimately.***

If you are emotionally invested in a chiropractor-- as patients often are -- and you are reluctant to view him or her as greedy or incompetent, then try this experiment next time you have an appointment. Ask him or her if subluxations can be detected or corrected as a means to solving your neck or back problems. If the answer is "yes," you have already learned that this is a red flag for a non-evidence- based practitioner. If the answer is "no," ask how often the chiropractor tells patients that manipulation is not indicated for their condition. In my practice I have found that at least every fifth patient will probably not benefit from or require manipulation. A chiropractor's answers to those two questions will tell you a great deal about the chiropractor's scientific standards and about his or her approach to health care.

Sometimes, because of the "touchy-feely" nature of chiropractic care, patients demand continuing spinal manipulation beyond a demonstrated need for it.

Barbara Gallagher[6] was in an automobile accident that left her with worsening leg and knee pain, lower back pain and a feeling of "heaviness" in her hips. She was referred to an evidence-based practitioner who initially treated her with exercise and socio-

---

[6] Not her real name.

occupational advice such as "wear high heels as little as possible" and "cross your legs at the thigh only when absolutely necessary." Barbara saw the practitioner regularly for about three weeks and she began to feel significantly better. About that time the practitioner told her she would not be needing regular treatments anymore. He gave her detailed instructions about continuing her recovery on her own. Barbara protested, insisting that she was not ready to terminate the treatments. The practitioner gently explained again why continued office visits were not in her best interest. Barbara finally understood that maintaining her regained well-being was largely her responsibility and that abdicating that role to the health care system would only leave her chronically dependent and ultimately a lot poorer financially.

Now that you have some idea of the difference in philosophy and approach between conventional chiropractors and evidence-based practitioners, take a quiz to see if you can identify which of the following health care professionals would have your best interest at heart. All of these stories are actual case histories, drawn from records of practicing chiropractors. Although some minor details have been changed, the evaluation process and course of treatment are presented here as described by the chiropractors themselves.

✔ Case #1: Marie, a 58-year-old female, had been treated by a chiropractor about ten years earlier for headache and low back pain. Her low back pain and headache had returned and she went to visit her chiropractor again on a Friday afternoon. That was a very busy time in the office. In a treatment room, she was given a basic range of motion examination. She was scheduled to come back the following week for a complete examination because she had not had one in so many years.

During the exam the chiropractor noticed that she had an unusual cough. Marie explained that she had been treated for eight months for bronchitis. After the chiropractor performed spinal manipulation on the patient in an attempt to relieve her head and low back pain, he instructed his technician to take chest x-rays. "As you are aware," the chiropractor wrote in a letter, "chiropractic offices are not 'qualified' to order anything other than spinal x-rays, but I felt that this was a serious problem that shouldn't be ignored."

While examining her x-rays the chiropractor noticed something. On the chiropractor's advice the series of chest x-rays was repeated at the offices of a medical doctor. Within ten days Marie was in a major hospital undergoing cancer surgery. Her visit to her chiropractor helped to detect the cancer and as a result, the early detection helped extend her life by approximately two years.

✔ Case #2: Brian is a 41-year-old male referred to a chiropractic office by his family doctor who had scheduled him for surgery on the left elbow. Brian was suffering debilitating pain and losing the use of his left arm. He had been diagnosed with tennis elbow and possible carpal tunnel syndrome.

At the chiropractor's office Brian's medical history was taken and he received an orthopedic examination of his left upper extremity as well as tests to rule out any cardiac involvement. Brian was treated seven times in two weeks with manipulation to the wrist and elbow. He also received tetanizing, which is constant low-volt current to the body. At the end of seven treatments he was completely pain-free and functional, and had cancelled his scheduled surgery. The chiropractor saw Brian about nine months later. Brian was still pain-free and had full use of his left arm. He had not undergone surgery, which would have been an expensive and probably unnecessary procedure.

✔ **Case #3:** Jessica is an 18-year-old female who was in a fairly serious automobile accident. For the first time in her life, she was experiencing back and neck pain. Her neighbor was a chiropractor and she asked if it was appropriate for her to make an appointment with him. He said he would be glad to try to help her. At the first visit the chiropractor took her history and performed an orthopedic examination. Although she had been injured he decided not to x-ray her because she was only eighteen and he did not want to expose her unnecessarily to radiation. The chiropractor instructed her about exercising to relieve the pain and performed spinal manipulation on her a total of five times. She had no pain after the fifth visit. She has not been back to see him since.

Did you figure out which case was treated most appropriately and with the best interest of the patient at heart? Several red flags may have gone up in your mind concerning Marie, our first patient. Was an updated history taken? She had not been seen in that office for years yet there is no indication that her medical history was brought up to date. Had that been done her eight-month bout with bronchitis would have been revealed right away.

Secondly, when the chiropractor noticed a cough that was severe enough for him to be concerned, why did he go ahead and perform spinal manipulation? Should he not have referred her immediately to her medical doctor?

Third, why did the chiropractor order chest x-rays even though he admits that a chiropractic office is not "qualified" to take chest x-rays?

Although it may seem like the chiropractor acted in the best interest of the patient because she lived two years longer (and there is no way to empirically prove that connection, by the way), he certainly was not acting in her best financial interest. The chest x-ray series alone may have cost her more than $100. The x-rays were completely unnecessary because they were taken again at the hospital.

For Marie, here is what should have happened: her medical history should have been taken as soon as she sat down in a treatment room. Upon learning of her extended fight against bronchitis the chiropractor should have directed her to see her physician as soon as possible. There should have been no manipulation and no chest x-rays in the chiropractor's office. That "something wrong" was detected by the Chiropractor may have gotten her some treatment for cancer sooner rather than later, it was a stroke of luck. A lot of chiropractors may have taken x-rays and noticed nothing unusual since they are not trained to detect cancer from x-rays.

Brian's story is a fifty-fifty proposition. True, he received a short, appropriate course of spinal manipulation that may have prevented a need for surgery. But he also received low-volt stimulation – tetanizing – an unproven remedy. In all likelihood Brian's problems would have resolved without the electrical stimulation.

I also wonder what "tests" were performed "to rule out cardiac involvement." A single test may have been appropriate because pain in the left arm sometimes can signal a heart attack, but since Brian had been under the care of a medical doctor and had been experiencing the pain for some time, even one test may not have been indicated. Besides, how qualified is the chiropractor to diagnose a heart problem?

Jessica's case was handled the most appropriately. Her medical history was taken, she was given an orthopedic exam, and she underwent a short course of spinal manipulation, an approach that has been clinically proven to relieve neck and back pain.

The Plural of Anecdotes Is Not Data

Now that you know something about what constitutes appropriate evaluation and appropriate treatment from a chiropractor, you may believe that testimonials from the patients of practitioners or from the practitioners themselves are an effective method of gauging whether you are dealing with evidence-based health care professionals. Or, you may believe that asking questions about their philosophy and approach will lead you to the information you need to make an informed decision about where to receive your medical care.

If you rely solely on testimonials or on a chiropractor's answers to your educated questions, you are probably short-changing yourself and your right to quality, clinically-proven health care. You need to recognize what other patients already have learned -- **your health is your responsibility.** I understand how burdensome that realization can become, when it is so tempting to lean on a health care professional for what you think are all the right answers. We need to acknowledge that health is not always found at the doctor's office, but disease is. If we want to stay out of the doctor's office as much as possible we have to actively maintain our health. When we get sick we need to participate fully in medical decision-making so we can boost our chances of being in control of our future.

Face-to-Face With Your Mortality, How Will YOU React?

Some medical doctors will tell you that when faced with chronic or life-threatening illness, patients tend to fall into three groups. The first are those who want the doctor to make all the decisions and tell them as little as possible, either about the course of the disease, the selected treatment, or the treatment's side effects.

The second patient group comprises the majority - those who want just enough information to allow them to feel somewhat knowledgeable about their condition. These patients are typically afraid to learn too much about their disease. That is because either they are worried they will not be able to interpret what they discover through books, medical journals, or the Internet, or they fear they will come across disturbing or depressing information.

The third patient group - and this is considered the rarest - is composed of those who are determined to become intellectual sponges. They need to know. They come to know their odds of survival and they learn about the effectiveness of every possible treatment option and every conceivable side effect of every treatment option. They scour published medical research for more answers and search out support groups.

While you may not be inclined to join the third group's exhaustive approach to finding answers ~ whether you are well or ill ~ I urge you to move progressively closer to a mentality that says you are in charge of your health.

Abdicating control over your health may leave you chronically dependent on caregivers. The treatment from caregivers may or may not be evidence-based. Relinquishing responsibility also will leave you much poorer financially, to say nothing of your pain and lack of well-being.

Brian was lucky. His course of treatment lasted only through seven visits, but because his chiropractor relies on unproven treatments, his experience *could* have been quite costly. Ensuring that you receive appropriate, evidence-based care is a two-way street. If you expect the health care professional to be competent and to interview you thoroughly, then you must actively participate in your own care. Passive physical modalities ~ such as electrical muscle stimulation, hot packs or ultrasound, i.e.: things that are done to you ~ usually do not work because they are often unproven.

In an article in *The Journal of Prosthetic Dentistry* published in November, 1998, author D.M. Brunette, Ph.D. notes, "The term 'quack' refers to those who boast and promote unproven remedies, whereas 'charlatans' are those who engage in fraudulent practices ... There is near general agreement that a good proportion of alternative practitioners believe sincerely in their therapies, and indeed such positive attitudes probably contribute to the placebo effect, which, in turn, aids treatment acceptance."

Ah, The Key Word: Acceptance

Author D.M. Brunette also points out, "The vast majority of unconventional therapies are not supported by controlled studies. Often, they rely on lower forms of evidence, *most specifically testimonials.* [italics added for emphasis]

"Textbooks on clinical investigational design view case studies are poor quality evidence for the effectiveness of any treatment," Brunette continues. "Testimonials in which individual persons attest to the effectiveness of a therapy should be considered as poorly described case studies... Testimonials should be ignored as a source of reliable information, particularly when presented by advocates with a vested interest in providing treatment."

Although Carl, Barbara, and Jessica received evidence-based care, it is not in your best interest to automatically assume that their chiropractors would provide the best care according to your medical needs. It is up to you to begin to figure out which kind of caregiver ~ a primary care physician, a neurologist, an orthopedic surgeon, or a chiropractor ~ is most ideally suited to addressing your particular situation. It is not an easy process but there are resources you can turn to make the task more manageable. Some of the better resources are presented in the appendix.

Here are two phrases you may want to remember when it comes to your health: "show me the data" and "what is the statistical probability?" If your chiropractor cannot produce the first or interpret the second, **then take my advice: find a new one!**

Chapter 6

Deciding Where To Take Your Pain

The exhaustion of passion is the beginning of wisdom.

--Anonymous

Please read the quote above again. Chances are you are reading this book because you are passionate about the kind of health care you receive whether it is traditional or alternative care. Enthusiasm for a particular way of doing things is wonderful, but we all know that emotion can cloud reason. So for the duration of this chapter I am asking you to set aside your passion and your bias. I want you to be as open-minded as possible about what you read here.

Did you know that as of mid-2001 Amazon.com offered 326 book titles on back pain, 71 titles on evidence-based medicine, and twenty (although twelve are out of print) on spinal manipulation? Not surprisingly, there is not a single book offered on evidence-based spinal manipulation.

From among just the titles related to back pain you can choose any of dozens of approaches: the McKenzie Method, the Mind-Body Connection, the Mendsendieck System, Backhab, Chinese Qigong, Prolotherapy, Source Completion Therapy, traditional Chinese medicine, aromatherapy, chiropractic care, complementary medicine, homeopathy or self-hypnosis. You can read *Back Care Basics, Mind Over Back Pain, Healing Back Pain Naturally, Back Pain Helpbook, Back Pain Bible, The Bum Back Book, The Back Pain Sourcebook, Back in Shape: A Back Owner's Manual* or *The Back Almanac. These are* among the hundreds of tomes available in exchange for your hard-earned cash.

Are any of these books the best source of information for ridding yourself of pain? If they are evidence-based, then they may be useful. If they advocate untested or unproven remedies ~ you can ignore the testimonials ~ you already know that they are not going to tell you what you need to learn.

There is one evidence-based booklet available on back pain. Called *The Back Book*, it is available only at **www.amazon.co.uk**, Amazon.com's

United Kingdom web site. Edited by Martin Roland and published in 1997, it contains the latest medical evidence and the best and most up-to-date advice on how to deal with your back yourself, recover quickly, keep moving, stay active, avoid disability, and help yourself to lead a normal life. Interestingly, there has never been a study in the United States that relies on this evidence-based back book. Hmmm.

Let us help you find a chiropractor who performs evidence-based spinal manipulation , which has been proven to be helpful in the treatment of acute low back pain in studies. You may think that because I have been tough on chiropractors throughout this book I am singling them out as non-evidence-based practitioners. I am zeroing in on them because, at their finest, they offer the best treatment option available for episodic back pain. Episodic back pain is not chronic or related to a medical condition that may require surgery. This treatment is also known as spinal manipulation. Ninety percent of all spinal manipulation is performed by chiropractors.

Unfortunately, you will have difficulty finding such a practitioner. As noted in Alternative Medicine and Ethics, edited by James M. Humber and Robert F. Almeder, only "a small percentage of chiropractors ... spurn unscientific practices, and confine their practice to musculoskeletal problems." That is a pity for chiropractors because right now, as I have said before, just three to ten percent of the adult population visits a chiropractor at some point in their life. If chiropractors chose to embrace their scope of practice and their area of expertise, then they could become so highly regarded that there would not be enough chiropractors in the world to handle back pain sufferers.

Several times I have referred to spinal manipulation for back pain as being evidence-based. Have you wondered where the evidence is? You can find some of it in a *Clinical Practice Guideline* booklet produced by the Agency for Health Care Policy and Research (AHCPR), part of the U.S. Public Health Service and the Department of Health and Human Services, in 1994. This is found in Appendix A, Useful Resources.

Why refer to a book published so many years ago? Because it was one of the first publications to study the effectiveness of various treatments for low back pain by painstakingly examining numerous randomized clinical trials for each type of treatment. An updated version of this valuable public service has never been issued. The chiropractic medical community was outraged by the conclusions of a 23-member panel and applied such pressure to AHCPR that the agency has never published such a booklet again.

In the publication called *Acute Low Back Problems in Adults*, the 23-member panel of health care professionals concluded that "manipulation can be helpful for patients with acute low back pain problems without radiculopathy [nerve pain] when used within the first month of symptoms." The panel based its finding on what it calls "moderate research-based evidence," defined as "one relevant, high-quality scientific study or multiple adequate scientific studies."

To put this in perspective realize that this advice to spend money on chiropractic care is based on perhaps a single study. Even if it is based on many studies, those studies are only of moderate value, based on the definition presented.

So you still may not be convinced that an evidence-based practitioner who performs spinal manipulation at appropriate times is what you need. Perhaps you have been to a chiropractor in the past ~ one who performed spinal manipulation the way it was intended ~ but your pain returned. Who else can you turn to? There are scores of traditional and alternative medicine practitioners you may be considering. Family physician. Orthopedic surgeon. Neurologist. Physical therapist. Acupuncturist. Herbalist. Homeopath. Naturopath. These are just a few of the options available to you. Friends, relatives, co-workers or neighbors may have shared stories about their "life-altering" experiences with some of these practitioners. The anecdotal evidence may be compelling, the attraction to a "magical cure" irresistible. Do not be a moth led to the flame. Anecdotal evidence could cost you several months' worth of house payments. Remember that in ninety percent of cases back pain will resolve on its own within six weeks of onset.

Granted, six weeks of pain is a long time and there is nothing wrong with investigating treatments and ways to remain functional in your daily activities. But you do need to think carefully about the treatment you are seeking. You also need to pay close attention to the particulars of your back pain. Do not ignore important warning signs.

Indications For Traditional Care:

Seeing your family physician is indicated if:

- Your back pain is accompanied by a fever, indicating an infection;
- Your back pain does not diminish even when you change positions, or it appears to be worse during the night, perhaps even waking you up with its severity;
- You have experienced significant trauma to your neck or back. The key word here is "significant." In that case, back pain may be sign of a fracture.

A referral to an ER or specialist may be necessary if these conditions are diagnosed.

There are times *not* to see an orthopedic surgeon or neurologist. Do not go see an orthopedic surgeon or a neurologist for simple mechanical back pain that will, in ninety percent of cases, resolve on its own within six weeks. A surgeon is trained to do surgery; a neurologist will consider organic causes of your pain. Do not waste the physician's time or your own seeing a specialist within the first four weeks of the onset of back pain when it is highly likely that basic strain is the cause. It is unnecessary and expensive, and it will not give you the results you want: simple relief from pain.

Is Physical Therapy The Solution?

When is it a good idea to go to a physical therapist? The answer depends on what approach the therapist intends to take. If he or she plans to use physical agents and modalities such as ice, heat, massage, ultrasound, cutaneous laser treatment (a hand-held light device used to treat acupuncture points on the skin), or electrical stimulation, then you may want to reconsider.

In *Acute Low Back Problems in Adults*, the panel of experts concludes that the use of physical agents and modalities in the treatment of acute low back problems yields insufficiently-proven benefit. The key point is this: the result of these treatments do not justify their cost. As an option, patients may be taught self-application of heat or cold to the back at home. The panel goes on to say that only two studies evaluated physical agents and modalities in patients with acute low back pain. Neither found significant differences in pain relief between patient groups receiving physical agents and modalities -- including flexion exercises (such as bending over to touch your toes) or extension exercises (standing straight up and placing your hands on the small of your back, then leaning backward) -- and groups receiving a placebo.

If, on the other hand, the physical therapist is stressing certain kinds of exercise, one or two visits may be helpful to learn the most beneficial routines. Here is what the panel says about exercise:

- Low-stress aerobic exercise can prevent debilitation due to inactivity during the first month of symptoms and thereafter may help to return patients to the highest level of functioning appropriate to their circumstances.
- Aerobic (endurance) exercise programs, which minimally stress the back (walking, biking or swimming) can be started during the first two weeks for most patients with acute low back problems.
- Conditioning exercises for trunk muscles -- especially back extensors (where you lie in a face-down position, bring your head up and arch your back as far as you can) -- when gradually increased are helpful for patients with acute low back pain, especially if symptoms persist. During the first two weeks these exercises may aggravate symptoms since they mechanically stress the back more than endurance exercises.
- Back-specific exercise machines provide no apparent benefit over traditional exercise in the treatment of patients with acute low back problems.
- Evidence does not support stretching of the back muscles in the treatment of patients with acute low back problems.
- Recommended exercise quotas that are gradually increased result in better outcomes than telling patients to stop exercising if pain occurs.

So, if a physical therapist wants to put you through a stretching routine for your back, now you know that this is not the most recommended course of action. But, if he or she wants you to get on a treadmill for twenty minutes three times a week, that approach is supported by clinical evidence. You now also know that if you have suffered from low back pain for more than two weeks, trunk-conditioning exercises such as "lat pull-downs" or seated rowing repetitions might help you feel better. Your destination is "activity tolerance," *not* under-activity or overzealous working out. You have to learn to tolerate some discomfort while you are getting better.

Chapter 7

Alternative Medicine Is Encroaching on The Back Pain Business

There's no business like show business!

~ Irving Berlin, from "Annie Get Your Gun"

Up to now we have talked about chiropractic and the medical community. It has probably come to mind to ask the question: what about other types of treatments such as acupuncture, or herbs, naturopathy, and homeopathy? You may have heard good or bad things about one or more of these. Let us take a quick look at each to see if they have make a good treatment for your pain ~ or a substitute for proper medical care.

Acupuncture: The sticking point of alternative medicine

The jury is still out regarding the value of acupuncture treatment for back pain. It is not going to be a surprise for you to learn that support for acupuncture as a remedy for acute low-back pain is largely *anecdotal*, not clinical. Alternative medicine was built on anecdotal evidence. What exactly is anecdotal evidence? It is evidence whose strength rests purely in stories and untested, random results. You may have friends ~ highly educated, professionally successful people who demand proof of effectiveness for other products or services they "buy" ~ who may swear by the "miracles" they experience with acupuncture. You may be tempted to try it for pain due to its growing level of recognition among mainstream medical practitioners. My feeling? Be very, very careful.

Anecdotal evidence can appear to be one thing but in reality be something entirely different. For me that is epitomized by an episode of the 1960s-era television show *The Twilight Zone* in which aliens land on earth and convince the planet that their only mission is to help mankind and that mankind can live a blissful, bountiful life on the aliens' planet. The aliens – tall, balloon-headed, skinny creatures, of course – have even written a manifesto, "How to Serve Man." But the earthlings learn – just as many are boarding the aliens' spaceship – that all is not as it seems. "How to Serve Man," we discover, is a cookbook.

If you do not want to become an appetizer for chiropractors or other alternative medicine practitioners, do not rely on anecdotal evidence to decide whether to visit a particular practitioner. Get the statistical facts whenever possible.

Alternative medicine got a big boost in 1992 when the National Center for Complementary and Alternative Medicine (NCCAM, part of the National Institutes of Health) was established. Since then numerous so-called "clinical trials" on the effectiveness of a variety of alternative therapies have been conducted. An NIH consensus panel of scientists, researchers, and practitioners said in November, 1997 that clinical studies have shown that acupuncture is useful by itself or combined with conventional therapies to treat, among other conditions, lower back pain.

Interestingly, a summary of clinical studies is found at **http://nccam.nih.gov/nccam/fcp/factsheets/acupuncture/acupuncture.htm#clinical** includes the words "lower back pain" but the body of the consensus report does not. Here is what the consensus report at **http://odp.od.nih.gov/consensus/cons/107/107_statement.htm#2** actually says:

> *"There is clear evidence that needle acupuncture is efficacious for adult postoperative and chemotherapy nausea and vomiting and probably for the nausea of pregnancy. Much of the research is on various pain problems.*
>
> *"There is evidence of efficacy for postoperative dental pain. There are reasonable studies (although sometimes only single studies) showing relief of pain with acupuncture on diverse pain conditions such as* ***menstrual cramps, tennis elbow, and fibromyalgia.*** [bold type is added for emphasis]. *This suggests that acupuncture may have a more general effect on pain. However, there are also studies that do not find efficacy for acupuncture in pain.*

> *"There is evidence that acupuncture does not demonstrate efficacy for cessation of smoking and may not be efficacious for some other conditions. Although many other conditions have received some attention in the literature and, in fact, the research suggests some exciting potential areas for the use of acupuncture, the quality or quantity of the research evidence is not sufficient to provide firm evidence of efficacy at this time."*

You can see that the words "lower back pain" are not in the "Efficacy for Specific Disorders" section of the report.

You may think because the government sponsors NCCAM, unconventional treatments now carry credence. They still do not and here is why: the studies upon which recommendations have been based often contain a faulty or illogical premise. For example, acupuncture is based on the theory of "meridians" that are defined as the fourteen pathways throughout the body for the flow of qi (pronounced "chee") -- or vital energy -- accessed through acupuncture points. Just like subluxations, no one has been able prove that "meridians" and "qi" exist. If researchers cannot prove they exist we have to ask the question: how can practitioners prove their treatments have any actual therapeutic benefit for their patients?

The National Center for Complementary and Alternative Medicine was established specifically to justify unconventional therapies, so naturally it issues collective opinions that support administering these therapies, at least in limited instances.

As Stephen Barrett, M.D., a well-known expert on medical fraud, notes in *Alternative Medicine and Ethics*, NCCAM was spearheaded by promoters of questionable cancer therapies who wanted more attention paid to their methods. Most of the advisory panel members have been promoters of "alternative" methods, and none of the center's publications have criticized any method.

So, even though these studies carry the apparent weight of government-sanctioned research, it is still considered junk science. Reputable studies are randomized clinical trials and the most objective evaluation of study findings comes from a meta-analysis of all randomized clinical trials that are attempting to gauge the effectiveness of a specific treatment. Many of the meta-analyses for alternative therapies are drawn from anecdotal evidence, not statistical or quantitative evidence. Evidence-based medicine routinely does not rely on consensus or expert opinion.

In Acute Low Back Problems in Adults, the panel says that a meta-analysis, based on 51 clinical studies on acupuncture used for various types of chronic pain including back pain, found that the quality of even the better studies was mediocre and their results highly contradictory. Specifically noted was that most of these studies did not provide an adequate control group or were not adequately blinded. "Blinded" means the subject does not know whether he or she is receiving a placebo or an actual treatment. None of the studies demonstrated an advantage of needling in the "appropriate" Chinese meridians over "misplaced" needling. The authors concluded that the efficacy of acupuncture for treatment of chronic pain remains doubtful.

Unless you enjoy spending money on unproven remedies, it may be in your best interest to skip the acupuncturist.

Can Herbs Help?

Herbalism is practiced by chiropractors, acupuncturists and unlicensed herbalists. With herbal treatments you consume herbs and they, hopefully, help you. You should know that many herbs contain potentially thousands of chemicals that have not been completely catalogued. Some herbs may be therapeutic, some may be toxic. Does it sound like a good idea to play Russian roulette with your health?

In addition, herbalists can be incredibly expensive. One visit could cost you well over $100. Does it make any rational sense to pay an unlicensed practitioner potentially hundreds of dollars just because your neighbor or your colleague has had good luck using herbal preparations? Remember the Placebo Principle. Up to 35 percent of people given a placebo as treatment get better *simply because they believe they will get better.* No research studies based on quantitative evidence have proven the effectiveness of herbalism in treating any ailment. Resist the temptation to be a sheep.

Homeopathy: If A Lot Is Bad, A Little Is Better

Homeopathy is based on a centuries-old notion that if large amounts of a substance can produce symptoms in a healthy individual, tiny amounts can cure diseases having those symptoms.

Jack Raso, M.S., R.D., in the *Dictionary of Metaphysical Healthcare*, says the major principles of homeopathy include: (a) A substance with specific effects in a healthy person can cure a person with similar symptoms. (b) The process of repeated dilution and vigorous shaking of harmful substances renders them "medically active" yet "free of side effects." (c) Each body has only one soul, thus a person has only one core problem at a time, and only one remedy is necessary for a "curative action." (d) Proper selection of a remedy requires taking into account numerous minutiae about the patient's situation. (e) "Mind symptoms" usually are more important than physical symptoms. (f) Humans are "soul energy" vibrating in an "energy pattern" (the so-called physical body). (g) Cures involve interaction of the soul and cogitative, affective, and physical processes. Usually "inner peace" is the first response to a remedy, "better energy" the second, and "physical" cure the last.

What does that explanation mean? If you understand it *and* can empirically demonstrate these concepts, then perhaps there is more to homeopathy than previously realized. How do you clinically verify "energy patterns?" Energy patterns, qi, meridians, subluxations -- do you see a pattern emerging? They try to explain why something works or does not work based on something that may not exist.

Naturopathy: The Science of One-Stop Shopping

According to the National Center for Complementary and Alternative Medicine, naturopathy views disease as a manifestation of alterations in the processes by which the body naturally heals itself and emphasizes health restoration rather than disease treatment. Naturopathic physicians employ an array of healing practices including diet and clinical nutrition; homeopathy; acupuncture; herbal medicine; hydrotherapy (the use of water in a range of temperatures and methods of applications); spinal and soft-tissue manipulation; physical therapies involving electric currents, ultrasound, and light therapy; therapeutic counseling; and pharmacology. Wow! All that from one practitioner?

This approach may sound appealing. It is far more soothing to think about "health restoration" rather than "disease treatment." If this is such revolutionary science, however, why are not allopathic physicians -- the medical doctors - rushing to become naturopaths? After all, they could bill you for far more services than just exams and consultations and they might just emerge heroic in the process. You already know the answer. Naturopathy is unproven, experimental, murky despite claims by naturopaths that thousands of modern clinical studies have validated a variety of natural medicines used by NDs. Echinacea for the immune system and St. John's Wort for depression are just two examples.

Alternative medicine practitioners ~ including a large sector of chiropractors ~ frequently suggest that a boatload of clinical studies support their work. The first question that should come to mind when you see these statements is, "When and where were any ten conducted?" If practitioners claim thousands of studies, then they should easily be able to cite ten. The second question that should come to mind in the face of such claims is, "In what peer-reviewed medical journals did these ten studies appear?"

Be suspicious of other ploys that alternative medicine practitioners use. Dr. Barrett gives fifteen examples in his book *The Vitamin Pushers: How the "Health Food" Industry is Selling America A Bill of Goods*. In the quotes that follow I have added my comments in parentheses.

- "We really care about you!" (Spoken like a true chiropractor)
- "We treat the whole patient." (As opposed to MDs, who ask you to cut off your head to be treated)
- "We attack the cause of disease."
- "Our treatments have no side effects." (ALL treatments have possible side effects in some people)
- "We treat medicine's failures." (Code for "get out your wallet")
- "Think positive!"
- "Jump on the bandwagon." (That is, be a sheep)
- "Our methods are time-tested." (The more time we spend with you, the more money you will spend with us)
- "Backed by scientific studies." (Show me the studies)
- "Take charge of your health!" (Get out your charge card and take a deep breath)
- "Think for yourself." (This underscores the whole point of this chapter)
- "What have you got to lose?" (Besides your time, money, self-esteem and confidence in the medical system?)
- "If only you had come earlier." (But since you did not, I am not under the gun to prove myself to you.)

- "Science does not have all the answers." (But does it have more than you do?)
- "Do not be afraid to experiment." (After all, you could be home exercising right now and planning a healthy meal, but instead you are here in my office willing to be my guinea pig because you are too lazy to do what's good for you.)

Think of all the money spent on alternative health care. Literally millions of dollars. This money could be spent on legitimate research into life-threatening diseases.

IOC Bans Austrians in Blood-Transfusion Case

Here is a case where an alternative medicine technique backfired, and rightfully so. Two Austrian cross-country skiers were disqualified and two team officials banned from the next two Winter Olympics over the use of blood-transfusion equipment at the Salt Lake City Games. A two-games ban was also handed to Volker Mueller, the German chiropractor who prescribed the blood treatments. Mueller told investigators he has been carrying out the treatments at his clinic in Germany for years, doing the same for other athletes from other countries.

The Austrians' claim that the blood treatments were merely for therapeutic reasons. The IOC considers any manipulation of blood as a form of blood doping, so the board ruled that the Austrians violated the Olympics' anti-doping code.

Will Simple Bed Rest Help?

So where, in the final analysis, should you take your back pain? There is one absolute answer: NOT to bed. According to *Acute Low Back Problems in Adults*, "prolonged bed rest for more than four days may lead to debilitation and is not recommended for treating acute low back problems."

It might be tempting to rest a lot when you have back pain. Resist the urge. Better yet, resolve to avoid back pain in the future. Start by recognizing that you are responsible for the health of your back and every other part of your body.

Good Health Will Take a Small Effort from You

It is so easy to turn over the responsibility for your own health to a perceived expert, instead of doing the often-difficult work needed to maintain good health. Your health depends on three factors:

1) genetics (which you cannot control),
2) lifestyle choices (Entirely within your discretion) *and*
3) the kind of medical practitioner you choose to see to keep or regain your health. (Choice is largely within your control.)

Genetics you cannot control The other two you can, and should.

Lifestyle choices have an amazing impact on your overall health. For example, if you are overweight, over fifty, and you rarely or never exercise, you may be a heart attack waiting to happen. If you throw smoking into that recipe for disaster, you could be looking at a heart attack or a stroke – not to mention lung cancer – under the age of fifty. When it comes to your health, the choices are up to you.

It is largely the same with the health care providers you see. When you choose a provider who practices according to evidence-based principles, you will be given appropriate advice or remedies, and you will get better sooner. If you elect to see a chiropractor, for example, for your back pain, he or she may tell you that you need 42 spinal adjustments and that in between adjustments you should rest as much as possible. It is a wonderful way to build a disability claim, is it not?

> ***Exercise – as a preventive measure and as a remedy for pain – is essential. It is so fundamental to good health that here is how I characterize it: put off exercise today ... welcome illness tomorrow.***

Or, as Mark Twain liked to say, "The only way to keep your health is eat what you don't want, drink what you don't like, and do what you'd druther not."

Ortho or Neuro Specialist?

If you go to your family doctor after about four weeks of pain and he or she recommends that you see a specialist because you have a herniated or ruptured disk, who should you go to next: an orthopedic surgeon or a neurosurgeon?

There are pluses and minuses to each specialty. I spent three years in a hospital working with orthopedic surgeons and I have interacted with neurosurgeons during eighteen years of private practice as a chiropractor. My opinion is that neurosurgeons tend to be more technically skillful than orthopedic surgeons, but orthopods generally are more committed to following up with you to make sure you are getting proper rehabilitation and that you are starting to restore function. My experience has been that when a neurosurgeon finishes your surgery, he is done with you save for a post-operative visit.

I tend to think that it is probably better to see an orthopedic surgeon unless you have especially complicated spinal issues, but be aware that your primary care physician probably will refer you to whoever he knows. That could be a neurosurgeon as easily as an orthopedic surgeon.

What if you have back pain that has lasted for more than six weeks? Where should you take your pain then?

> ***Maybe you have already been to your family doctor. After four weeks you could not bear the pain a moment longer. Your doctor ruled out an infection, a tumor, a fracture and even a herniated disk. She told you that most likely you have mechanical back pain. The advice? Go home and exercise gently.***

But now it is two weeks later and the pain is unrelenting. To whom should you turn?

If you go to a chiropractor you could be in his or her clutches for months. Like many alternative medicine practitioners, chiropractors are highly reluctant to refer their patients to other practitioners. Alternative medicine is the black hole of health care: any patients that touch the outskirts of their practice can get sucked in forever. Academically, many alternative practitioners believe they can offer you the panacea, so why would they refer you to someone else?

Your objective is not just to rid yourself of the pain. Your goal is to prevent your acute back pain from becoming *chronic* pain. While acute pain can be helped by a short course of spinal manipulation and exercise, there is nothing out there that has been proven to help long-lasting back pain except continued exercise, a trip to a health resort, and hiring a team of health care professionals to try to figure out what is wrong with you.

Can you guess the chief cause of back pain progressing from acute to chronic? It is job satisfaction, or rather dissatisfaction. If you hate your job, would it not be great to be able to claim disability from chronic back pain? But if you are experiencing actual unrelenting back pain, time away from work is not going to salve your job-related unhappiness.

It is important to understand that chronic is different from recurring pain. If you get relief from acute pain for even a short time, then you do not have chronic pain. With chronic pain you never get a break.

If you are still experiencing back pain at six weeks after onset and you have already been to your family doctor, then it is time to see ~ drum roll, please ~ **a psychologist**.

A psychological evaluation is the recommended course of action for back pain heading into chronic mode when there are no known organic or anatomical cause. Find out how your emotions are influencing your spinal column. I am not suggesting that you are mentally ill or that something is fundamentally flawed in your psyche. I am saying that we are learning more and more about psychological influences on back pain and about how psychology often has more of an impact on the severity and duration of back pain than anatomy or physiology does. Keep an open mind about what your mind is trying to tell you.

But okay, you just have episodic back pain that started ten days ago. Should you see an evidence-based practitioner who will perform a limited course of spinal manipulation?

> ***Yes, you may want to consider seeing someone who performs spinal manipulation only in one limited circumstances: if you have low back pain. For mid- and upper back pain, wait to see if the pain resolves on its own.***

If you have low back pain, how do you find a reputable, ethical practitioner who happens to have spinal manipulation in the arsenal? You will find out in the next chapter.

But before you turn the page, consider this:

D.D. Palmer, the founder of chiropractic in 1895, is reported to have said, "Your spinal column supports three things: your head, your neck, and your chiropractor."

Chapter 8

Selecting A Chiropractor Who Can Help You

Knowledge will forever govern ignorance and people who will mean to be their own governors must arm themselves with the power which knowledge gives.

--James Madison

Protect yourself from becoming a gravy train for an unscrupulous practitioner.

If you are among the ten percent of the population that takes the alternative care crapshoot and will continue to visit a chiropractor, or you are considering a first visit for whatever reason, this chapter is definitely a "must read" for you. After what I have talked about in the previous chapters, you may be thinking that the term "honest chiropractor" is an oxymoron. To some degree that is true. But there are ways to improve your chances of finding a practitioner who has bothered to read, understand, and acknowledge evidence-based medicine.

Rule 1:

Get Off The Mis-Information Superhighway

It is easy to be overwhelmed by the avalanche of claims, counter-claims, and promises made by chiropractors. You will find the misinformation nearly everywhere you look: newspaper and magazine ads, and articles, books, direct mail pieces, the telephone, the Internet and particularly, the yellow pages of your phone book. In one large metropolitan area alone, where fewer than 1,000 chiropractors are in practice, you can look at sixteen pages of advertisements for chiropractic services! If you were to rely on the yellow pages alone to find a chiropractor, how could you even begin to narrow your search beyond geographic area? They are all crying "NOOPE!" (No Out of Pocket Expenses). Due to "ethical" concerns, NOOPE lately has been replaced by No Out of Pocket Costs. You will also see an offer of "free x-rays" but then in smaller letters you will see "if medically necessary" or "if indicated." That is because it is unethical to give away free ionizing radiation. Many ads also boast of "free initial consultations." NOTHING – especially in the world of chiropractic – is really free of charge.

When you view these advertisements objectively you begin to see how chiropractic offices use loud, colorful ads to reel in patients just as if new patients are the catch of the day. "STOP THE PAIN!" one half-page ad proclaims in inflamed red type. "NEED RELIEF?" another asks, then indicates that the office will treat neck and shoulder pain, lower back and leg pain, auto and work injuries, *and* provide family care.

Chiropractors are typically listed under "Physicians–Chiropractic" Is it sad to think about someone in pain, not understanding the true nature of chiropractic care, thumbing through the yellow pages to find a doctor who they believe can literally rub or snap their pain away? How frightening it must be to have as your only resource a phone book full of multi-colored ads that nearly jump off the pages with confusing, misleading statements.

You do not have to be a fish. Remember these few simple facts about chiropractic advertising in the telephone book:

- A full-page color ad in the yellow pages can cost between $2,500 and $3,000 a month! Someone has to pay for this.
- Since most offices generally are not very busy, they can justify an ad by plans to recoup its costs through protracted treatment recommendations.
- A fancier ad, a larger ad does not indicate anything better. What it does indicate is the chiropractor must ultimately produce more money.
- "A Palmer graduate" simply means the chiropractor has graduated from Palmer Chiropractic College in Davenport, Iowa. Because the institution's identity contains the last name of the founder of chiropractic – D.D. Palmer – you are supposed to be impressed. Frankly, no chiropractic education should impress you. Remember, the majority of chiropractors have not even graduated from a four-year undergraduate college.
- Do not get carried away by lots of initials after a chiropractor's name, such as DC, MS, CCSP, CICE, CIFCME or DABFP.

Most of these suggest certification of some kind or another or that the chiropractor has additional training, but the alphabet soup does not necessarily mean the chiropractor does not believe in subluxations. In the same spirit do not be swayed by "diplomat in..." In traditional medicine a diplomat is a physician qualified to practice in a medical specialty by virtue of advanced training and experience in the specialty, followed by passing an intensive examination administered by a national board of senior specialists. In chiropractic a diplomat is a practitioner who takes courses through a chiropractic college once a month. It does not allow them to provide any types of treatments superior to a chiropractor who does not have diplomat status.

The bottom line: Never let advertising ~ especially phone book advertising ~ be the source of your office choice. Do not even open the phone book to look for a chiropractor. Ideally the chiropractor you eventually select will not be listed in the yellow pages anywhere, though some may just to keep their name in a public domain.

Rule 2: Know What Professional Memberships Are and What They Mean to You

Where do you turn to find a professional? For chiropractic professionals, the first place you can look is the National Association of Chiropractic Medicine (NACM) web site, whose address is **www.chiromed.org**. Read about the organization's demand that its members ascribe to scientific principles, not to a "theosophy." The organization describes theosophy as a belief in an unproven hypothesis.

Members of NACM must sign a statement rejecting most of what conventional chiropractors believe in. "The first and foremost requirement for membership in the NACM is that a Doctor of Chiropractic Medicine ***renounce*** the chiropractic hypothesis and/or philosophy; that is, the tenets upon which their scope of practice is based" The introduction on the web site goes on to state "The original chiropractic hypothesis, stated simply, is that 'subluxation' is the cause of 'dis-ease'...[T]he term 'subluxation' has never been defined by the profession in a way as to have universal acceptance within the chiropractic profession."

To find out if there is a member of the NACM in your area send an email to the manager of the NACM web site. Identify your city and state and request the name of a chiropractor near you who is a member. Because only twenty to thirty percent of chiropractors belong to any organization at all, it is unlikely that there is an NACM member in your city, but any NACM referral is far safer than any word-of-mouth advice, any advertising claims, or any testimonials.

Why do so few chiropractors belong to professional organizations compared with the vast majority of medical doctors who choose to affiliate with at least one industry-oriented organization? The answer lies partly in the fact that chiros cannot agree on a consistent way of responding to patients' needs. There is a saying that if a lone chiropractor were stranded on a desert island, he or she would need at least two professional organizations for support because of the enormous disparity in viewpoints.

Chiropractors often do not have the money for organizational dues. And, in the case of the NACM, why would they want to join a group that will limit the scope of their practice? From a chiro's point of view it is pretty ridiculous to join a professional organization when there is no universal agreement on what chiropractors should be doing to help the patients who come to them.

Rule 3:

Know The Two Main Types Of Chiropractors

The chiropractic profession cannot agree on what a subluxation is or is not, nor can it find common ground for the services a chiro should offer. Chiropractic is populated by what are known as "straights" and "mixers."

Although it may sound like we are talking about sexual orientation, "straights" and "mixers" are actually the two most common types of chiropractors that you can encounter. A "straight" chiropractor is more likely -- if he or she belongs to any organization -- to be a member of the International Chiropractors Association. "Straights" use only those methods of examination, analysis, and "adjusting" whose objective is correcting "vertebral subluxation."

A "mixer" is likelier to be a member of the larger American Chiropractic Association. This type of chiropractor typically wants to reduce or eliminate disease or its symptoms, and may use spinal manipulation in addition to ultrasound, diathermy, electrical muscle stimulation, nutritional counseling, homeopathy and hair analysis -- and the "fix of the week."

> ***The only evidence-based association for chiropractors is the National Association of Chiropractic Medicine. Any other chiropractic organization exists to promote its membership.***

You probably will have to go beyond Rules 1, 2, or 3 to find a chiropractor.

Rule 4: Look to Those With Experience

...and I am not talking initially about the experience of your friends. Remember, that is anecdotal and should carry only minimal weight. Everyone likes their doctor particularly if they only know one. I am talking about contacting a managed care organization. If you have an HMO or a PPO, then start by looking in the provider directory. There may or may not be listings for chiropractors. If there are, you know that these practitioners at least have met minimum professional standards and have jumped through one or two ethical hoops in order to qualify as plan providers. It is still not an optimal way to pick a chiropractor but it is better than relying on neighbors, co-workers, and friends. These should be your absolute last option.

You can see that finding an evidence-based chiropractor can be a monumental undertaking. I am not entirely certain that I have convinced you of the importance of insisting on an evidence-based practitioner.

That was the situation with a friend of mine. We had discussed these topics numerous times in the past. She had gotten relief from a chiropractor before and has educated, highly intelligent friends who have been delighted by homeopaths, herbalists, and naturopaths. So I offered her a challenge:

Find one chiropractor who follows evidence-based guidelines for treatment of back pain.

I suggested we try three scenarios. In each she would explain her "condition" over the phone to the chiropractic office. In addition, she developed a scenario of her own. In all she called eight chiropractic offices and spoke directly with five chiropractors.

***Scenario #1:** In this scenario she calls to explain her condition: "I've had low back pain with pain shooting down my leg for two weeks. The pain moves farther down the leg all the time; right now it is almost down to my toes."*

Remember readers: evidence-based guidelines say that **spinal manipulation is not appropriate for back pain accompanied by nerve pain.**

Here is the chiropractors' responses:

✔ Chiropractor #1: "You're experiencing nerve pressure and nerve weakness caused by a misalignment of your spine. We can correct this mechanical problem through adjustments."

✔ Chiropractic office #2: "This is definitely a problem that a chiropractor can solve. It's probably caused by your spine being out of alignment."

Summary: It sounds like they want to get her into their office doesn't it?

***Scenario #2:** "I've had a dull, constant pain in the mid-back region for three weeks. Regardless of what I do the pain never goes away. In fact it gets worse at night. Changing positions does not help, exercise does not help, anti-inflammatory medications do not work."*

Remember readers: these are **tumor-like signs and symptoms.**

✔ Chiropractor #3: "You have a misalignment of your spine. That bone has to be put back in place. An adjustment is a gentle, pleasurable experience."

Being fair, we gave the chiropractor an opportunity to reconsider his recommendation: We added:

"My friend's mother had these same symptoms about two years ago and she ended up being diagnosed with cancer."

The chiropractor's answer: "That's a possibility, I suppose, but it's very unlikely."

Very unlikely? We just gave this chiropractor some pretty precise symptoms of cancer, and he says "very unlikely."

Scenario #3: "I woke up this morning with severe back pain. I am running a fever, I am sweating profusely, the back of my head hurts terribly, and the symptoms seem to be getting worse."

Remember readers: these are **symptoms of infection**, which demands immediate medical attention.

✔ Chiropractor #4: "I really think chiropractic will help you. I am not one of those who doesn't like MDs, I'll tell you that right up front. My family goes to MDs. There are times when MDs are important. But in this case I think chiropractic can help you. In my heart of hearts I believe that."

Whoa! Red flag! *Why does he have to trust his heart? What about scientific evidence?*

✔ Chiropractor #5: "We'd certainly welcome you to come in and see us, or you can go to your family doctor or the ER first."

...the emergency room first?? Doesn't that indicate the chiropractor recognizes that this could be serious?

✔ Chiropractic office #6 (our caller says she had already been to her own chiropractor and had gotten no relief): "If you've already been seen today, I doubt very seriously that another chiropractor could help you."

How about telling the patient to go see a medical doctor?

✔ Chiropractic office #7: "You may have an infection. You should see a doctor first."

Okay, the chiropractor answered correctly. We found <u>one</u> chiropractic office that provided her with sound advice.

On this next scenario, remember that there is no evidence that chiropractic care is indicated for **neck pain**.

Scenario #4: "I woke up this morning with neck pain. Is it appropriate for a chiropractor to treat neck pain?"

✔ Chiropractor #8: "Oh, absolutely."

Thee is no need to comment about Chiropractor #8 -- "absolutely!"

The Key Point Is...

...You would not ask a chiropractor to heal your gallbladder or manipulate away a dental cavity. You would not do that because you know that there are scientifically-proven treatments for these situations. These scientifically-proven treatments are administered by qualified doctors who rely on the latest evidence presented in peer-reviewed clinical literature, not to mention the years and years of medical school. So why would you accept any chiropractic practitioner's *promise* to "adjust away" your back or neck pain?

Here is why: the natural course of back pain is six weeks or less *when you do nothing but continue your normal routine.* Remember that nine out of ten back pain cases resolve on their own within six weeks. Sigh, but we live in a quick-fix society where we are impatient and anxious to return to "normal." Interestingly, we are often willing to tolerate pain in other parts of our bodies - afraid, for example, that an on-again, off-again pain in our abdomen might be something serious- - and we ignore it or hope it goes away. When we are confronting back or neck pain, however, we rarely think it is life-threatening, so we focus on getting relief. There isn't the fear that the care-giver is going to tell you your going to die.

Conventional medicine cannot offer instant help, usually, but nearly everyone has experienced or knows of someone who has experienced relief from back or neck pain at the hands of an alternative practitioner. Complementary and alternative medicine providers -- CAM providers - are successful only when they treat minor conditions, not serious illnesses. Alternative medicine makes a living and develops a reputation by practicing its theosophies in the gray zone of health care. A CAM provider will not cure cancer, magically repair a broken bone, or reverse kidney failure. But he or she can eliminate back pain under the right circumstances. Through a combination of the Placebo Principle -- where you think you will get better, then you will - and the natural history of such pain, a CAM provider has a very good chance of making you feel better. What a deal. You could have seen a psychologist for that.

Rule 5: Watch Your Wallet

There are a lot of ways a practitioner can get at your wallet. They can scare you into accepting a big hit by convincing you that expensive treatments are necessary, perhaps implying that you are a fool for not accepting their "human" overtures. Or they may try to nickel and dime you -- selling you things you do not need like icepacks, x-rays, supplements, and their "fix of the week." Show your smarts by saying "No, I don't want to overdo it *because after the appropriate spinal manipulation I'll be feeling better already*." You'll also be feeling better because you escaped with your lifesavings intact, or you have kept in the good graces of your health insurer by saving them a lot of unnecessary expense.

Making Your Appointment

We have established that locating a scientifically-based chiropractor is the biggest obstacle to getting good care. Now, as an educated consumer, you know what to watch out for -- the playing field has been leveled -- and you can insist on receiving appropriate care for your low back pain from the chiropractor, and forget the "way out" remedies. You just have to know the red flags to watch out for, the right questions to ask, and the correct responses to questions.

Once you have decided to seek help from a chiropractor and have selected the one least likely to rip you off, you are going to call for an appointment.

These do's and don'ts give you a reasonable chance of seeing a chiropractor who will provide you with a short, affordable course of appropriate spinal manipulation.

<u>DO</u>:

- Since there is no such thing as a chiropractic emergency, and you know that it is truly lower back pain, wait 72 hours -- about three days -- before calling for an appointment. This lets you see if your low back pain goes away on its own. Even if it does not go away within that time, undergoing a spinal manipulation within the first three days of the onset of pain is usually not recommended. Your joints and ligaments may be in the acute phase of healing, and if so, that is too early to benefit from a manipulation.

- **Stay as active as possible** while you are waiting to see if the pain goes away on its own, or while waiting for the appointment with the chiropractor.

- **Ask if the chiropractor restricts his practice to complaints of the spine**. If the answer is "no" or "he does a little bit of everything" or "yes, but he also does acupuncture, nutrition counseling, and hair analysis" or if you hear dead silence, then hang up the phone immediately.

- **Ask if the chiropractor performs spinal manipulation only by hand**. An evidence-based chiropractor will not use electrical muscle stimulation machines or spring-loaded mallets or ultrasound to treat your back pain. Do not go to a chiropractor unless you are assured that spinal manipulation is done only by hand.

- **Tell the receptionist or chiropractor that you have no insurance of any kind – but that you can and will pay. Stress that you have not suffered any type of injury**. You can tell them about the injury after he appointment is set. You are less likely to be targeted for long-term chiropractic care when you do not have insurance or when an injury is not involved.

<u>DO NOT:</u>

- **DO NOT seek chiropractic care for anything other than low back pain** that you have had for more than 72 hours and less than one month. If your pain is present anywhere else such as the neck, upper back, or mid-back above the bra-line, or if you have had low back pain for more than four weeks, then consult a general practitioner.

- **...DO NOT accept or be persuaded by arguments** that chiropractic care is appropriate for other pain near the spine or other ailments. Manipulation of the neck can be particularly dangerous.

- **...DO NOT take your children to see a chiropractor ~ ever.** Chiropractic care for children under six is not recommended by the NACM. If your child is under thirteen, chiropractic care should occur only in conjunction with a pediatrician's guidance. This is very important so I must be redundant here concerning children and chiropractic. The Alberta Medical

Association in Edmonton, Alberta cautions: "Chiropractic use of x-rays in infants and children to diagnose so-called vertebral subluxations is unscientific and of no value whatsoever. Without any benefit to the child, these x-rays can contribute to the risk of cancers and genetic damage. Parents should never allow their children's spines to be x-rayed by a chiropractor." The organization also says: "There is no scientific evidence whatsoever that so-called chiropractic spinal adjustments result in any correction of the child's spine. These adjustments are ineffective and useless."

- **...DO NOT rest or go to bed any more than you usually would** no matter what a chiropractor tells you. Staying as active as possible is critically important to resolving back pain quickly.

Rule 6: Insist on Full Disclosure

Now you are in the waiting room on the day of your scheduled appointment. On the clipboard of papers they give you to fill out, look for two items in particular: an informed consent form and a fee schedule.

Do not fill out any other forms until you determine whether an informed consent form is part of the package. This document represents the ethical obligation of any practitioner to indicate in writing treatment risks, treatment benefits, possible results if no treatment is administered, and alternative approaches to your problem. The informed consent form is the form most people simply glance at and sign. In this situation it is particularly important to READ IT CAREFULLY. The form should be between one and three pages in length and should contain phrases such as "A chiropractic adjustment of your neck can cause a stroke" or "an adjustment to your mid-back can cause a fractured rib" or "spinal adjustment to your low back may cause a herniated disk." **If no risks of treatment are listed, then the office does not believe in full disclosure.** You can ask the receptionist "where is the form that explains the risks?" but I would return the clipboard and leave immediately.

Here is the Informed Consent Form I use in my office.

INFORMED CONSENT FORM

PATIENT NAME: ____

You are to read this INFORMED CONSENT FORM. Once you have read and understands the statements presented here, you may sign this form on page 2. If you do not understand the statements here, do not sign this form. We will answer any questions you have BEFORE you sign this form, and before any treatment is considered or begun.

The primary treatment used by doctors of chiropractic is the spinal adjustment. I will use that procedure to treat you.

The Nature of the Chiropractic Adjustment

I will use my hands upon your body in such a way as to move your joints. That may cause an audible "pop" or "click," much as you have experienced when you "crack" your knuckles. You may feel or sense movement.

The Material Risks Inherent In Chiropractic Adjustment

As with any health care procedure, there are certain complications that may arise during a chiropractic adjustment. Those complications include: factures, disc injuries, dislocations, and muscle strain, Horner's Syndrome, diaphragmatic paralysis, cervical myelopathy, and costrovertebral strains and separations. Some types of manipulation of the neck have been associated with injuries to the arteries in the neck leading to or contributing to serious complications including stroke. Some patients will feel some stiffness and soreness following the first few days of treatment.

The Probability of Those Risks Occurring

Fractures are rare occurrences and generally result from some underlying weakness of the bone, which we check for during the taking of your history and during examination and x-ray. Stroke has been the subject of tremendous disagreement within and without the profession with one prominent authority saying that there is, at most, a one-in-a-million chance of such an outcome. Since even that risk should be avoided if possible, we employ tests in our examination that are designed to identify if you may be susceptible to that kind of injury. The other complications are also generally described as "rare."

Ancillary Treatment

In addition to chiropractic adjustments, I intend to use the following treatments:

____

____

These treatments involve the following additional significant risks:

____

____

The Availability and Nature of Other Treatment Options

- Self-administered, over-the-counter analgesics and rest
- Medical care with prescription drugs such as anti-inflammatory muscle relaxants
- Hospitalization with traction
- Surgery

INFORMED CONSENT FORM **Page 2**

The material risks inherent in such options and the probability of such risks occurring include:

1. Overuse of over-the-counter medications produces undesirable side effects. If complete rest is impractical, premature return to work and household chores may aggravate the condition and extend the recovery time. The probability of such complications arising is dependent upon the patient's general health, severity of the patient's discomfort, his or her pain tolerance, and self-discipline in not abusing the medicine. Professional literature describes highly undesirable effects from long-term use of over-the-counter medicines.

2. Prescription muscle relaxants and pain-killers can produce undesirable effects and patient dependence. The risk of such complications arising is dependent upon the patient's general health, severity of the patient's discomfort, hit or her pain tolerance, self-discipline in not abusing the medicine, and proper professional supervision. Such medications generally entail very significant risks -- some with rather high probabilities.

3. Hospitalization in conjunction with other care bears the additional risk of exposure to communicable disease, iatrogenic (doctor-induced) mishap and expense. The probability of iatrogenic mishap is remote, expense is certain, exposure to communicable disease is likely with adverse result from such exposure dependent upon unknown variables.

The Risks and Dangers to Remaining Untreated

Remaining untreated allows the formation of adhesions and reduces mobility, which sets up a pain reaction, further reducing mobility. Over time, this process may complicate treatment, making it more difficult and less effective the longer it is postponed. The probability that non-treatment will complicate a later rehabilitation is very high.

DO NOT SIGN UNTIL YOU HAVE READ AND UNDERSTAND THE ABOVE.

PLEASE CHECK THE APPROPRIATE BLOCK ([ ]) THEN SIGN BELOW:

I have read [ ] or have had read to me [ ] the above explanation of the Chiropractic Adjustment. I have discussed it with Dr. Preston Long and have had my questions answered to my satisfaction. By signing below I state that I have weighed the risks involved in undergoing treatment and have myself decided that it is in my best interest to undergo the treatment recommended. Having been informed of the risks, I hereby give my consent to that treatment.

____________________ _________________________

dated printed name

____

signature

Witness

____

____________________ signature of parent or

printed name guardian (if a minor)

____

signature of witness

If an informed consent form meets the standard, then make sure a fee schedule is included in the bundle of forms.

There should be a single fee schedule. The price range for services should be something like this:

- **Consultation/Exam/Report of Findings: $30-$40**
- **Spinal manipulation: $15-$45**
- **Exercise education/counseling: free (or should be!)**
- **X-rays: $30-$40 per film**

Exercise education should be included as part of any treatment. If the chiropractor wants to charge you for that, leave. Remember that *you* do not want to have x-rays at the chiropractor's office. X-rays should only be taken at a medical doctor's office or at a hospital, however it is acceptable to list x-rays on the fee schedule because it is within clinical guidelines to take x-rays after four weeks of unrelenting low back pain.

If any other services are listed such as nutrition counseling, hair analysis, electrical muscle stimulation, acupuncture, then you may run. This is a red flag to indicate a non-evidence-based practitioner.

Keep in mind that the lower the fees the greater the chance that repeated visits will be recommended.

If either the informed consent form or fee schedule is missing from the clipboard, go to the receptionist and ask for those forms. If the office does not have these forms or there is any hesitation on the part of the office staff to give them to you, my recommendation is that you choose to leave right then and there.

Do not ever be ashamed to leave. Other people have left this office before and others will leave in the future. You may even do what a friend did, explaining as they handed back the clipboard, "I have got to be home to receive a very important phone call."

Let us assume that the informed consent form meets the standard and that the fee schedule lists only reasonably priced services appropriate for a chiropractor to offer. Now we move on to the next form on the clipboard. It is a general questionnaire asking you questions about your health status today and about the history of your health.

At the bottom of this form you will probably be asked to select the level of care you want. You can typically choose from statements like these:

- treat me just long enough to get me out of pain
- treat me to correct and stabilize the problem
- treat me according to the doctor's recommendations

Many people will choose the last statement, risking a personal disaster by believing that the chiropractor is knowledgeable about spine problems and has the best interest of the patient at heart. **Do not select the statement that resembles the third choice**. You may end up paying for hundreds of dollars' worth of treatments you do not need. *Choose the statement that most closely resembles the first option.*

You will also find a form that contains a drawing of a human figure. This form will ask you to indicate with X's where your pain is located and how severe the pain is. Be honest. Do not exaggerate your pain. Being honest and not exaggerating will decrease your chances of the chiropractor making long-term care recommendations.

Rule 7: Bring Along a Healthy Dose of Skepticism

Now you are ready to meet with the chiropractor. **Bring along a healthy dose of skepticism**. He or she routinely spends more time with you than any other practitioner. Some studies have shown that the consultation by the chiropractor is more important to resolve your symptoms than the actual treatment given. Typically, after the introduction, you will be asked how long you have been experiencing your problem, what your symptoms have been, and what measures you have taken to control the pain. You will probably find him or her charming, personable, and warm. That is to build your confidence in them. You may find yourself impressed by talk of "restoring function" or "alleviating nerve pressure" or "improving the quality of your life." Do not let this language lull you into agreeing to costly or unnecessary treatments. If you hear words like "subluxation" or "bone out of place" instead of words like "mobility," then do not accept care. It is a red flag and you can and should choose not to accept their care. Be on your guard; you are dealing with a practitioner who makes his living in the gray zone of health care. Polish your radar, burnish your skepticism before you even step into the office. There are no universal principles in the world of chiropractic. It is up to you to don a detective hat in pursuit of truth. It is all about your health care and not about padding their bank account.

The first consultation should take about half an hour. What you tell the practitioner during this consultation should determine the level ~ or thoroughness ~ of the physical exam.

Regardless of the level of the physical exam, **the first thing that should occur** is assessment of your basic vital signs: temperature, pulse, and blood pressure. The chiropractor probably also will examine your back to determine the extent or limitations of your functional abilities.

Do not accept recommendations for x-rays unless a fracture, tumor, or infection is suspected. A single x-ray series of the lower back delivers to the gonads the equivalent radiation of a chest x-ray every day for six years. You do not need x-rays from the chiropractor. The total exam should take about half an hour.

Ideally, the practitioner will present a report of findings to you at that **first visit.** That is his or her conclusion about the origin and severity of your problem, based on the consultation and the exam. Also, ideally, you will receive a spinal manipulation of your low back at that first visit. The first appointment should last less than an hour and one-half, including advice about exercise.

All this should cost less than $100. The practitioner should not recommend that you come back for more than two or three additional appointments. Your second appointment, if scheduled, should be at two to three days after your initial visit. The best approach is to urge you to call the chiropractor's office at forty-eight hours ~ two days ~ if you are still experiencing significant pain. At that point you can make a second appointment. You can expect to feel about 85 percent better after your first visit. Within two weeks, I tell my patients, they will not remember my name.

By your third and, we hope, your final visit, the chiropractor should be educating you about the importance of exercise and continued activity, and about factors that can aggravate back pain ~ poor posture, women wearing high heels, etc. The goal is to keep you OUT of the office.

Remember These Additional "Don'ts"

Do NOT buy any cold packs, ice packs or heating pads from a chiropractor. First of all it is a conflict of interest for a practitioner to recommend such physical modalities and then try to sell you the products needed to employ those modalities. If a medical doctor prescribed Amoxicillin, a common antibiotic, and then tried to sell it to you himself, wouldn't your radar go up?

Secondly, and perhaps most important, physical modalities such as ice or heat often do nothing for back pain. If the chiropractor tells you to apply heat or ice at any point during treatment, thank him for the advice and go on your way without buying anything.

Do NOT accept a recommendation for maintenance care. Remember what I said in Chapter 2 about chiropractic adjustments creating dependency? Continual or ongoing care is not indicated in the arena of chiropractic medicine. As G. Douglas Anderson, a chiropractor in Brea, Calif., noted in *Dynamic Chiropractic* in 1999, "It is high time we admit there is nothing conservative, holistic or natural about endless care, creating addiction to manipulation, or making unsubstantiated cure-all claims. On the contrary, an excellent argument can be made that the variety of tricks, techniques, and claims still used by a large percentage of our profession to keep fully functional, asymptomatic people returning for care is fraudulent. I wonder how long it will take for our profession to realize that over-utilization not only damages our reputation, but also costs us millions of dollars of business per year in lost referrals."

There are people who will never, ever go to a chiropractor for fear of over-treatment.

Results of a survey published in the January, 2000 issue of the *Journal of Manipulative Physiology and Therapeutics* reveals that 95 percent of those chiropractors responding to the survey agree that maintenance care ~ MC ~ minimizes recurrences of problems. Another extremely high percentage- ~ 90 percent ~ believes that the purpose of maintenance care is to optimize health. Nearly as many – 88 percent- ~ believe that maintenance care prevents conditions from developing. The conclusion of the study is that despite educational, philosophic, and political differences, U.S. chiropractors come to a consensus about the purpose and composition of maintenance care. They believe that it is of value to all age groups and a variety of conditions from stress to musculoskeletal and visceral conditions. **This strong belief in the preventive and health promotion value of MC motivates them to recommend this care to most patients.**

But, more and more of the public can see right through this.

Is Chiropractic Against Your Religion?

Have you noticed how many times the words "believe" and "belief" are mentioned in conjunction with chiropractic care? Why are belief systems not reserved for religions? Unless you have already decided to follow the tenets of a religion that determines how you will receive health care, do you really want a belief system masquerading as a medical discipline dictating the kind of care you receive? Or do you want scientific evidence determining the appropriateness of your medical care? Would you want your surgeon recommending that you come to his or her office every week or month for the rest of your life post-operatively to have your knee bathed or massaged just because he "believes" it will prevent another torn meniscus? Would you not ask for the scientific evidence behind that recommendation or would you be happy with "This is simply what all orthopedic surgeons *believe* is in the best interest of a knee-surgery patient"?

You may be saying, "Yes, but traditional medicine's track record is not perfect either." Certainly not. In situations where there is no clear path to take many doctors use their best judgment or their instincts, or even their beliefs or experiences. But that is the exception not the rule. Treatments have a much higher rate of efficacy in medicine because they are born of clinical evidence. In chiropractic, relying on scientifically validated principles is a rarity. Nearly all chiropractic treatments are based on belief, judgment, or instinct. Remember my friend called a chiropractor who said, "In my heart of hearts, I *believe* that"?

Would it bother you to think of a chiropractor as a clergyperson? If the answer is "yes," then why would you accept and pay for non-scientifically proven recommendations from a health care practitioner? A chiropractor's office is not where you should be looking for a blending of medicine and religion.

> ***No matter how logical a chiropractor may make maintenance care sound, nothing is in actuality logical if it emanates from an unfounded or faulty premise. The doctrine of maintenance care springs from an erroneous foundation: that your problem will come back if your spine is not routinely and regularly adjusted.***
>
> ***Remember this, too: extraordinary claims require extraordinary evidence. If you are a doubter, then you do***

not have to prove to the practitioner that a recommendation, point of view, or course of treatment is NOT scientifically valid. It is up to the practitioner to prove scientific validity to you. Insist on that proof.

Absolutely do NOT agree to bring in your children, spouse, or pets for "free consultations." Beware of any chiropractic office that boasts "Small and large animal chiropractic" or "Dedicated family care" or "Gentle, effective care for newborns to seniors" among a host of other similar slogans. Keep in mind specifically how chiropractic can be beneficial with a short course of spinal manipulation for acute low back pain. Keep in mind that chiropractic is not at all appropriate as a preventive measure for disease or pain, and that it is not appropriate for children – anyone under age. Do animals need chiropractic care? Because they walk on four legs, they do not suffer low back pain. Care for animals and children is on the increase due to managed care limiting chiropractic visits. Simply, the chiropractor needs more patients and they do not care who or what those patients are. If your child needs a visit to a provider, choose a pediatrician. If you feel that your pet needs care, see a veterinarian.

Rule 8: Protect Yourself – The Exam

Do not be bamboozled by a chiropractor or any other medical practitioner. Do your own research and keep in mind these principles of truth advanced by famed astronomer Carl Sagan *(my comments are in italics)*:

- Wherever possible, there must be independent confirmation of the facts. *(A virtual career death knell for chiropractors.)*
- Encourage substantive debate on the evidence by knowledgeable proponents of all points of view. *(The key word here is evidence. Do not bother to debate courses of action for which there is no evidence of efficacy.)*
- Arguments from authority carry little weight. (*The word "authority" is used a lot in the media and has been scooped up by alternative medicine practitioners to lend credence to their claims.)*
- Try not to get overly attached to a hypothesis just because it is yours. (*Many chiropractors – by credo- – are married to their hypotheses).*

- If there is a chain of argument, every link in the chain must work. *("Subluxations cause pressure on nerves. Spinal adjustments can repair subluxations and eliminate that pressure." Where is the proof that subluxations, which is at the foundation for this assertion, exist?)*

Now, let us rate your exam.

There are tests and examinations that are appropriate and some that are not appropriate for an evidence-based practitioner to perform. Remember: the evidence-based practitioner is trained in chiropractic care. A chiropractor who is mindful of the best interests of the patient should, during the patient's first visit, go through the same steps as an orthopedic surgeon, a neurologist, or a neurosurgeon. First, the chiropractor should take a detailed case history. You will find that some do not. An evidence-based practitioner understands that most of the time spent in his or her office should be spent talking about your past, because as much as 95 percent of the patient's diagnosis is determined through the patient's history. Yes, 95 percent! As Hippocrates said, "Declare the past, diagnose the present." If the chiropractor does not sit with you for at least ten to fifteen minutes asking you questions about all aspects of your physical condition and your medical past, then you will know that, chances are, you are not in the presence of an evidence-based practitioner.

At some point during the visit your vital signs – height, weight, blood pressure, pulse, body temperature, respiration rate – should be checked. During the actual exam, your reflexes, sensation, posture, and range of motion should be assessed. There may be other components to the physical exam. Ideally, the entire visit transpires in a sequential manner The history determines the elements of the physical exam and the results of the exam determine whether any special testing – such as an MRI scan, a CT scan or blood work – should be ordered.

The X-Factor: X-rays ... A Very Real Danger

X-rays generally are warranted during the initial visit only when the history reveals that the patient has experienced a significant injury or may be suffering from an infection or a tumor. If the patient is complaining of low back pain or neck pain, for example, but has not suffered an injury, contracted an infection, or developed a tumor, it is not routine to expose the patient to ionizing radiation when there is no suspicion of these maladies. Only bones are seen on a conventional x-ray. Soft tissues such as muscles, ligaments, and tendons are not visible. X-rays should be taken of patients without these conditions only after about four weeks from the first visit, and only if the problem is not resolving. The vast majority of back and neck pain cases resolve within four to six weeks.

If the chiropractor says at the first visit that he or she would like to take an x-ray to rule out a subluxation, say good-bye as quickly as possible. The chiropractor is not practicing evidence-based medicine. Remember: "subluxations" have never been proven to exist. X-rays should not be substituted for an orthopedic exam.

...Free To Administer Almost Any Therapy They Wish – Or Can Get Away With!

By law, design, and definition, chiropractors are free to administer almost any therapy they wish. You will often hear about or see a chiropractor dispensing nutrition advice, selling vitamin therapy, performing acupuncture, aromatherapy, ultrasound therapy, or electrical muscle stimulation, and applying ice or heat to an area in pain, in addition to performing manipulations. Is there any scientific or clinical evidence that these approaches address patients' problems? The blunt simple answer is no. The value of any of these approaches has yet to be proven. Just because a chiropractor is legally able to deliver nearly any type of care does not mean the care is appropriate or evidence-based.

> ***What an evidence-based chiropractor is most qualified and trained to do is dispense advice concerning the importance of remaining physically active. He is also qualified to prescribe endurance exercises for you to work on at home. He is qualified to deliver a short course ~ one to three visits ~ of spinal manipulation.***

Chapter 9

The Kindly Giant's Guide to Back Care

Nature, time and patience are the three great physicians.

—H.G. Bohn

While reading the last chapter I hope it occurred to you that the best thing you can do for back pain is prevent it from occurring in the first place, and by taking practical advice that costs you nothing you can learn how to move, stand, exercise, and live in a way that helps your back, not hurt it. How about that for a great advertisement? Let us see if this chapter measures up to my claims.

Author and syndicated columnist Dale Dauten dubbed me "The Kindly Giant." Dale came to see me for his recurring back pain. He had been in search of an answer for his continually achy back and was happily surprised when I told him his back was healthy. He also was happily surprised to learn that I would not be recommending treatment after treatment to help him. He had finally found someone who was using evidence-based medicine to make a diagnosis and develop a proper treatment.

So far in this book we have seen how many chiropractors and other complementary and alternative medicine providers – CAM providers – will try all varieties of pseudo-logic, soulless promises, and bogus, scientific-sounding claims to entice you into paying for medical care that you do not need and that could actually harm you. Spinal manipulation as a remedy for neck pain, for example, can in certain instances lead to stroke. Regardless of what your symptoms may be, some chiropractors will insist on manipulating your neck. Do not let them.

Do Not Let This Happen To You!

There have been several examples cited in scholarly journals and consumer media of people who have had their necks "adjusted" or manipulated even when they had no pain there and then suffered a stroke. A Canadian woman went to a chiropractor for pain in her low back, yet her neck was adjusted twenty-one times! She had a stroke and became permanently disabled. In February, 1998, a twenty-year-old woman from Saskatchewan sought treatment for a stiff neck. After neck manipulation by the chiropractor, dissection of a vertebral artery interrupted blood flow to her brain. She lapsed into a coma right there in the chiropractor's office and died 24 hours later. Similarly, a young mother of four in Seattle suffered a stroke immediately after a chiropractic neck manipulation. She survived but still has difficulty with everyday tasks.

By now, you know the answer to this question: what is the best treatment for simple mechanical pain such as a sore neck? *Nothing.* The chances are you slept wrong. Your neck pain probably will go away within a week. Do not be swayed by convincing-sounding arguments from any CAM provider that you need treatment for your neck, whether or not you have pain. You especially do not want or need spinal manipulation.

> ***Whether you are experiencing neck pain, back pain, joint pain, or a headache ~ or any other kind of musculoskeletal pain ~ you do not need to and, in fact, should not seek alternative or complementary medical attention for at least three days.***
>
> ***Remember that conventional medical care is indicated immediately if you suspect a bone fracture, if you have a fever, or if you have pain going down your leg.***

It is important under those circumstances to be evaluated by an evidence-based practitioner ~ preferably a medical doctor. The doctor is likely to perform a diagnostic triage where he or she places you into one of three categories of back pain: 1) mechanical; 2) root (nerve) pain; 3) serious pathologies, such as cancer or infection.

The reason you want to see someone who practices evidence-based medicine and diagnostic triage is to reduce or eliminate practice variation, which is seen frequently in the CAM community. True evidence-based practitioners rely on the approach that has been scientifically demonstrated to be the best treatment for a particular ailment. For evidence-based providers, consistent patient care is a centerpiece of their practice.

Do-It-Yourself Treatments ~ A Guide To Self-Directed, Inexpensive Symptom Control

...away from a provider's office

Absent an injury that could have caused a bone to break, or absent any tell-tale signs of infection, there is plenty that you can do at home for yourself to ease your symptoms. These techniques cost next to nothing and rely on materials you probably already have on hand.

More than ninety percent of the time, whatever treatment you choose, you are going to get better anyway. Your goal is simply NOT to make things worse. Unfortunately, however, the problem does get worse in many instances when chiropractors and other CAM providers over-diagnose and over-treat and as a result contribute to chronicity ~ your continued pain.

As 21st-century Americans, it is difficult to assume responsibility for our own health care, because *passive* care ~ care which is done to us ~ *seems* more legitimate somehow, more grounded in clinical principles, more proven as a remedy. We would rather trust someone we perceive to be an expert because we have lost our ability to trust our own instincts. For example, does it not seem logical that application of ice or heat would alleviate pain? Your instincts tell you "yes." But throughout these pages I have been cautioning against letting a chiropractor administer cold or heat therapy. I have warned you not to buy a cold or heat pack from a chiropractor. Yet your common sense says "cold or heat or both has always helped pain." So what gives?

Your perception about the benefits of ice and heat are 100 percent correct. So why would you pay someone else to administer a treatment that is so easy for you to provide for yourself at no cost? Why would you pay someone to tell you that ice and heat can relieve pain? Is the pain relieved to a greater extent when a treatment as simple as this is delivered by someone other than you? The biggest problem with ice massage being delivered in a clinic is that it creates dependency and that can contribute to chronicity. If the only time you feel better is when you are in someone else's care, how will you ever escape the cycle of dependency?

The opposite of passive care is, of course, *active* care, which simply means caring for yourself. That is why I must continue to urge you not to let a chiropractor ~ or any other provider ~ talk you into paying for ice or heat massage. Clinical evidence suggests that managing musculoskeletal pain particularly in its early stages is a do-it-yourself project. **We have to**

accept active care whether or not we are comfortable with it or even like it. It is simply the best thing for a patient. And you can be proud of yourself. You did it!

Invest in yourself by not investing in unproven therapies. Take the money you would have spent on a chiropractor or other CAM provider, then do something inspiring, wise, or fun with it.

Time For Special Attention

> ***This is a very special section. What you are about to read is the core of this whole book. It is the most important information I can present to you, the guardian of your own health and well-being.***

Taking responsibility for your own health care may not be what everyone else is doing but it is the very best way to manage back pain. This approach will improve all of your symptoms associated with simple mechanical back pain.

Here are some steps you can take to minimize low back pain in particular -- where fractures or infection have been ruled out -- from the moment of **onset until 72 hours** have passed:

- Give yourself positive messages. I know that sounds very "New Age-y" and non-evidence-based, but research has demonstrated that encouragement is the single most important thing that a doctor can give a patient to stimulate an optimal chance for recovery. So give yourself the encouragement a doctor would give you. "There is nothing to stress about." "Backache is extremely common." "A full resolution of my problem will take only days to weeks" and "I will keep going on with my life and the pain will be gone before I know it" are some effective messages to repeat to yourself. As evidence-based chiropractor Craig Liebenson has noted, "The main cause of acute back pain becoming chronic is due to the patient taking on a sick role instead of viewing it as a temporary illness."

- Take a small Styrofoam cup and fill it with water until it is about two-thirds full. Put the cup in the freezer. After it freezes solid, peel the cup away until the ice is exposed. Then massage your pain with the ice for thirty to ninety seconds. Instant symptomatic control! This technique may not totally eliminate pain, but it probably will relieve it at least a little. You should regain some motion that was restricted by the pain. Doesn't this approach make far more sense than paying a chiropractor $50 or $60 to lay an ice bag on your back and then try to sell it to you when you leave?

- Consider what is known as the "Cadillac" of home care -- ice and moist heat rotations. Here is how they work: take a beach towel, wet it thoroughly, wring it out and put it in the microwave oven for 20 or 30 seconds. After checking that the towel is not scalding hot, apply this heated towel to your pain for five minutes or so. Then apply the ice for about one minute. After that reapply the heated moist towel for another five minutes. You may want to try three cycles of this method per hour.

- Take a non-steroidal anti-inflammatory medication. This is also known as an NSAID. You can buy these over the counter; they have names like Alleve, Tylenol, Motrin. Personally I like the active ingredient in Alleve because you can take one dose and it typically lasts for twelve hours. A therapeutic dose of the medication is ideal. Check with your family doctor to make sure a therapeutic dose is okay for you. Ask a pharmacist what the therapeutic dose is for the pain reliever you typically use.

- Do exercises that encourage flattening of the spine, such as lying on your back (1) and bringing your knees up to your chest (2), or a pelvic tilt, where you begin by lying on your back with your knees bent and your feet flat on the floor. Place your fingertips underneath your lower back. Contract your abdominals to tilt your pelvis so that your lower back presses slightly against your fingers. These movements flatten the low back curve and take strain off the region.

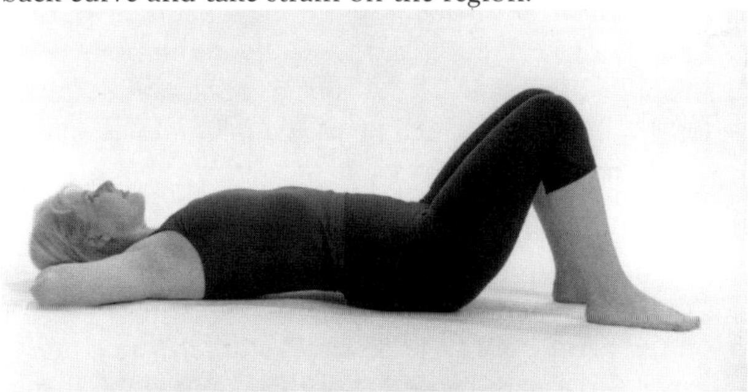

1.

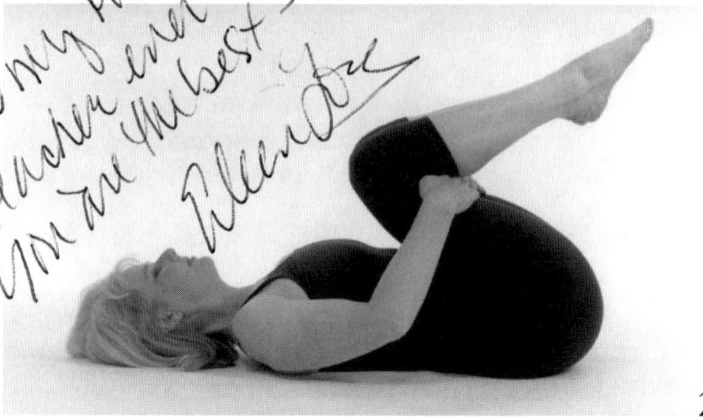

2.

- Do not wear a back brace. When movement is restricted, muscles can atrophy very quickly. A back brace can give you a false sense of security.
- Do not rest any more than is normal for you.

Here is what you should be doing for low back pain **from four days to two weeks after onset**, in addition to ice/heat applications as needed and taking NSAIDs...

- Remain as active as possible. Toward the end of this period, begin low-stress aerobic activity. The single best aerobic activity for low back pain is walking on a treadmill. Do not incline the surface of the treadmill; your walking speed is determined by tolerance of discomfort. I am asking you to use common sense here. It is not possible for me to recommend a certain walking speed for you because only you know how much pain or discomfort you can bear. Expect some discomfort. The walking speed you select should allow you to complete a twenty-minute session without groaning in pain. You should aim for a feeling of stretching your lower back muscles and ligaments, *not* a feeling of stressing them. Also, remember that your objective here is not cardiovascular fitness; the result of this exercise might be otherwise. The idea is to get blood pumping into your low back muscles, which helps you maintain as much mobility as possible. Take it very easy.
- If you do not have access to a treadmill, try regular walking. It's very important that you choose your walking surface wisely. Your first choice is dirt or grass. A high school track or a path on the perimeter of a park would work. If you must walk on a paved surface, asphalt is better than concrete. A better choice is

an indoor track surface, such as a polished wood floor. Your very last choice is concrete. If you have no choice but to walk on a sidewalk, it may be better to wait until you can find a dirt or grass path. The constant pounding that comes from striking your foot on concrete repeatedly is almost as detrimental as not exercising at all.

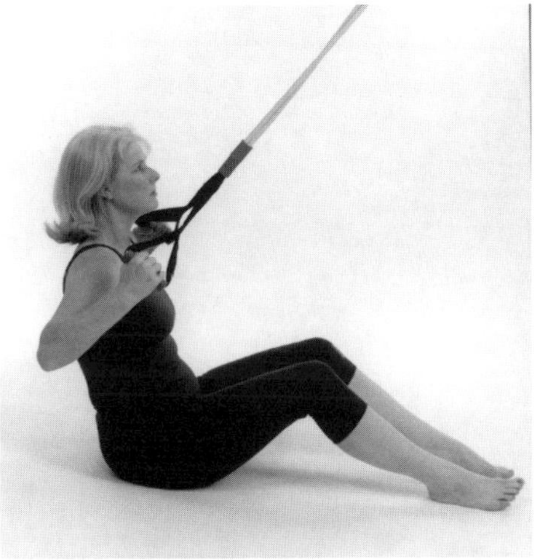

- To avoid chronic pain, right now is the time to start doing endurance exercises. My favorites are lateral pull-downs. This is any exercise where a bar with handles or surgical tubing is over your head and you pull the mechanism down to your chest.

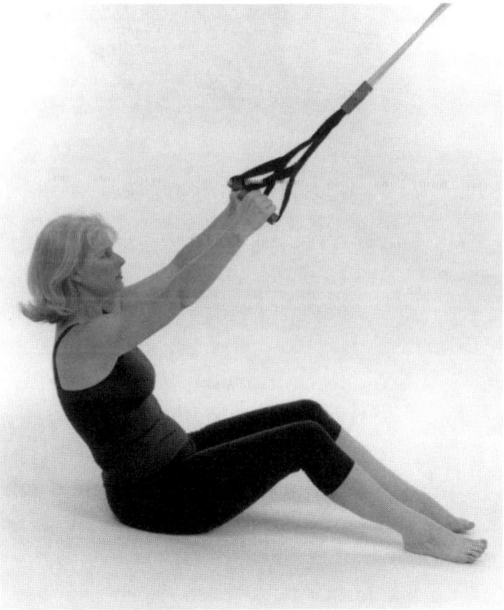

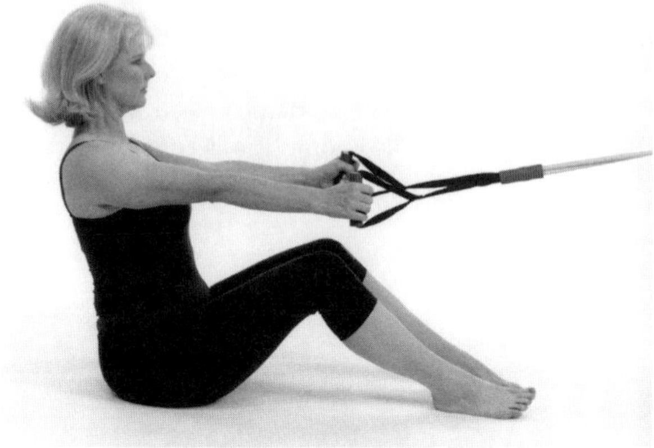

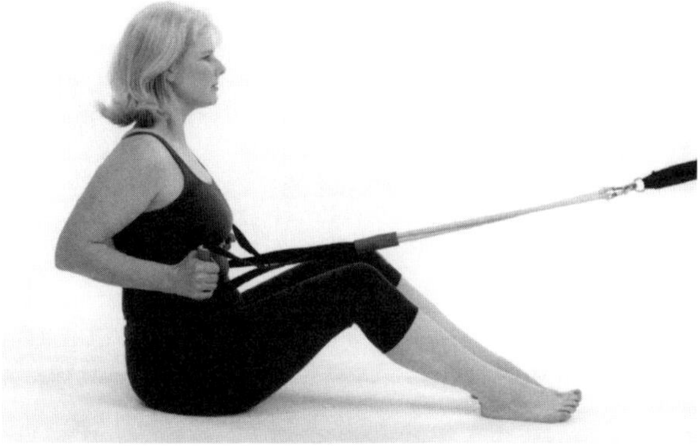

- Other favorites are seated rows ~ pulling a weighted bar or anchored tubing toward you.
- Another favorite is one-armed rows (pulling a dumbbell toward you from a bent-torso, drop-arm position). In any of these low-impact exercises, try various levels of low-to-moderate resistance to determine what is comfortable for you. The objective here is to train your muscles to support you during a normal day, not to build them up like a football player's. Think of the thigh of a marathon runner versus the thigh of a football player. You are also aiming for relatively low weight resistance and a high number of repetitions. Try to do three sets of 15 or 25 repetitions of each exercise at low weights.

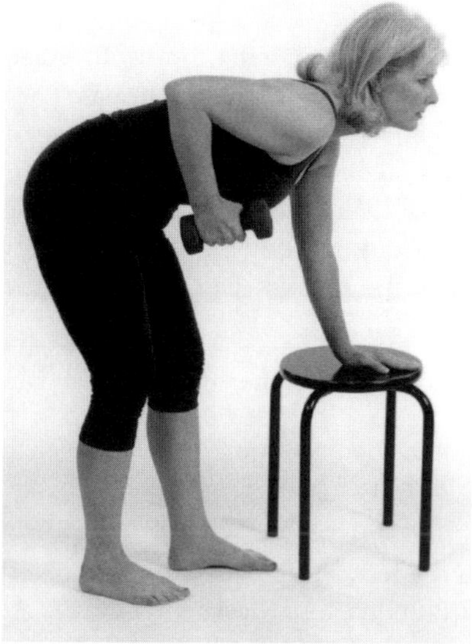

1. one-armed rows start position.

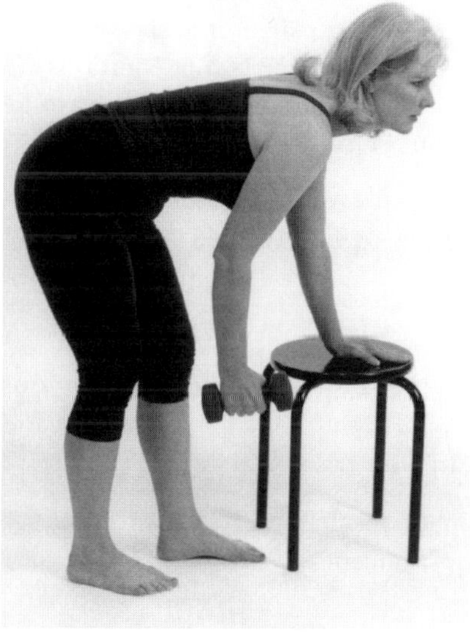

2. one-armed row finish position.

Remember: virtually no specialized equipment is needed. You do not have to go to a gym to perform these exercises. For lat pull-downs and seated rows you can use surgical tubing, which is available at any pharmacy. A can of vegetables can be used in place of a dumbbell.

During this phase of pro-activism, most people's pain diminishes significantly. It has been my professional experience that by day fourteen 85 percent of people with back pain will be completely functional. They will not necessarily be out of pain but they will be taking care of themselves and going about activities of daily living. Because pain is subjective and can vary greatly we do not look at pain or lack of it as the measurement of success. Rather we look at how well the patient functions in spite of the pain. Obviously, the less pain you have the more effectively you can function.

Here is what you could do from two to six weeks after the onset of pain whether or not you still have pain:

- Continue with your low-stress aerobics and endurance activities.

It is possible that you will be among the ten percent of patients who still have significant pain and restricted mobility four weeks after onset. At the four week point, further diagnostic work-up is indicated. This may include x-rays, reassessment and/or consideration of emotional issues. In Chapter 6, one of the best places to take your pain if it is six weeks old or older is to a therapist of your choosing. It is possible that emotions are preventing us from ridding ourselves of back pain. This is nothing to be ashamed of, but it is something we should be able to handle.

The International Association for the Study of Pain defines pain as "an unpleasant sensory and emotional experience associated with actual *or potential* tissue damage." The italics in that sentence are mine, added for emphasis.

What I tell my patients is this: If you are **still not feeling better in four weeks,** after using home remedies, performing low-stress aerobics, and taking pain relief medication, there are four possible reasons:

- The original diagnosis of simple mechanical back pain was incorrect. The wrong diagnosis meant the treatment was wrong, too.

- You have stayed so active that you did yourself more harm than good.

- You have not been active enough, or maybe you have been resting too much.

- Psychological issues are causing your pain.

If Pain Persists, Then Manipulation Is Not the Answer

Have you noticed that throughout this discussion of what you could do for back pain I have yet to mention spinal manipulation? That is because spinal manipulation is a passive modality not an active one. With back pain, active treatment is almost always better than passive treatment. If you are still in pain during the three to fourteen-day period after its onset, then it is far better to spend time, energy, and money on finding an evidence-based practitioner who can help you than it is to go to a typical chiropractor for a spinal manipulation.

Preventing Back Pain

The vast majority of us will suffer from back pain at least once in our lives. Back pain is so common that it is nearly unavoidable. What we want to avoid are recurrences of this pain and chronicity. We are looking to minimize frequency, intensity, and duration of pain. The war on back pain is one we will never win. That is, there is no guarantee against a chance injury. But you cannot afford to lose the war on back pain, so we work toward a state of equilibrium ~ a natural balance. A stalemate is a victory for the spine.

In an ideal world you do what you need to do to keep your back from aching in the first place. Here are twelve steps you can take to head off back pain before it starts:

1) Lose weight or maintain your normal weight. For every ten pounds of additional breast or abdominal weight you carry, you add 100 pounds of stress to the supporting soft tissue structures of your spine.

2) Increase abdominal strength. It is important that along with your back exercises you perform abdominal exercises to keep the musculoskeletal system in homeostatis, or balance. Do crunches regularly to build up those muscles but do not do sit-ups.

3) Avoid footwear such as cowboy boots and high heels that can offset the pelvis and lead to low back pain.

4) If you are on the telephone a lot and you frequently try to perform another activity while talking such as typing, cooking, bathing a child, etc., then use a headset instead of the

telephone receiver. This prevents you from craning and straining your neck.

5) Drink plenty of water. You have heard and read this advice in many places. Staying hydrated applies just as much to preventing head, neck, and back pain as it does to nourishing all of your other systems. Dehydration can lead to headaches.

6) When you travel take your own pillow. Even if you are at a bed and breakfast in Oconomowoc, Wisconsin – or anywhere – insist on a firm mattress.

7) Avoid flat-footedness when standing or sitting. Always raise one foot higher than the other. If you are at the sink doing dishes, open the cabinet under the sink and place one foot inside. That might feel awkward at first but it will take pressure off of your lower back. When you are seated, place one foot on a dictionary-size book, the other on the floor.

8) When seated, only cross your legs at the ankles when both feet are on the floor, or cross your legs ankle to knee. When you cross your legs thigh to thigh you increase your chances of back pain *and* varicose veins.

9) Lift heavy items only in the "safety zone" -- between your shoulders and mid-thigh. If you have to squat, bend, or reach to lift something, get help if at all possible. You do not want to risk weeks of pain for thirty seconds of impatience or carelessness.

10) Use common sense when trying to lift anything over your head. A woman reaching over her head for a ten-pound sack of potatoes has a greater chance of injuring her back than with almost anything else she can do. Even the lightest weight above your head can become very heavy. A five-pound weight above your head is equal to fifty pounds at chest level.

11) If you have any hint of back pain, *avoid* flexion rotation activities such as golf, bowling, vacuuming, or getting groceries out of the trunk of your car. Any time you are bending over and turning your body you are increasing your risk for a spine injury. Since golf and bowling are often chosen activities and vacuuming, putting away groceries and other activities of daily living are usually unavoidable, it is important to do two things: be faithful to all of the other steps in this list to minimize the

chance for back pain, and pay attention to the signals your body sends you. The morning you wake up with a mild backache is *not* the day to schedule a golf game.

12) Avoid tobacco. Smoking has been shown to decrease blood flow to the spine and to predispose one to osteoporosis. It is become such an issue that some members of the American Academy of Orthopedic Surgeons might refuse to perform spinal surgery on patients who are still smokers.

P-A-I-N-E-D

I know it is not politically correct to suggest that YOU are responsible for what happens to you. But I am asking you to be an adult and assume responsibility for your own musculoskeletal pain. Here is a simple acronym to help you remember how to recover from mechanical back pain: P-A-I-N-E-D.

Pain in your back usually is not serious

Attitude and positive messages are important

Ice and moist heat applied at home can be helpful

NSAIDs can relieve discomfort

Exercise is vital

Do not forget common sense...*You were born with some. Exercise it more, too.*

Another way to look at it might be evidence-based chiropractor Craig Liebenson's Four R's to Recovery. They are:

- **Reassurance.** This starts on the first day of pain. It will help you dispel the notion that your spine may be severely damaged.
- **Relieve pain.** He calls for home care strategies, NSAIDS, and spinal manipulation. (*My cautions: consider spinal manipulation only if you have been in pain for at least three days and less than a month and then only if the pain is in your lower back.*)

- **Re-activation.** This includes low-stress aerobics, endurance exercises and avoiding additional bed rest.
- **Rehabilitation.** This is physical training--focused, continued exercise--to avoid chronicity. *Following an exercise program, however simple, helps you.*

Someone once said that "only dead fish swim with the stream." Unfortunately, I can offer you no magic pill or no easy answers. Swimming against the stream is sometimes the only way to protect yourself, and that is especially true in the world of complementary and alternative medicine.

Again I have to mention that you should make every effort to avoid being taken in and sold something that I know does not work. Do not be lured in by so-called health-care providers' empty promises. If you want consistent good health and quality of life, then you have to invest time and energy in yourself. Notice I did not say money. Think of yourself as your own Home Depot for lifestyle remodeling, or that you are redecorating a new you inside and out. You have all of the tools available to you to avoid chronic back pain and to avoid being taken advantage of by non-evidence-based providers.

And, now that you have finished this chapter, you understand how you are in control of your health, your destiny, your life. I want to underscore that taking care of yourself is not rocket science, it is not a mystery, and it is not difficult. All it takes is a little practice and dedication.

Here is what the Agency for Health Care Policy and Research has to say in their published guideline, offered free to the public, on acute back pain. This is there most requested document ever. It is reprinted here as a public service, for your information.

Understanding Acute Low Back Problems

Patient Guide

Consumer Guideline Number 14
AHCPR Publication No. 95-0644: December 1994

About the Back and Back Problems

The human spine (or backbone) is made up of small bones called vertebrae. The vertebrae are stacked on top of each other to form a column. Between each vertebra is a cushion known as a disc. The vertebrae are held together by ligaments, and muscles are attached to the vertebrae by bands of tissue called tendons.

Openings in each vertebra line up to form a long hollow canal. The spinal cord runs through this canal from the base of the brain. Nerves from the spinal cord branch out and leave the spine through the spaces between the vertebrae.

The lower part of the back holds most of the body's weight. Even a minor problem with the bones, muscles, ligaments, or tendons in this area can cause pain when a person stands, bends, or moves around. Less often, a problem with a disc can pinch or irritate a nerve from the spinal cord, causing pain that runs down the leg, below the knee called sciatica.

Purpose

This ... is about acute low back problems in adults. If you have a low back problem, you may have symptoms that include:

- Pain or discomfort in the lower part of the back.
- Pain or numbness that moves down the leg (sciatica).

Low back symptoms can keep you from doing your normal daily activities or doing things that you enjoy.

A low back problem may come on suddenly or gradually. It is acute if it lasts a short while, usually a few days to several weeks. An episode that lasts longer than 3 months is not acute.

If you have been bothered by your lower back, you are not alone. Eight out of ten adults will have a low back problem at some time in their life. And most will have more than one episode of acute low back problems. In between episodes, most people return to their normal activities with little or no symptoms.

This booklet will tell you more about acute low back problems, what to do, and what to expect when you see a health care provider.

Causes Of Low Back Problems

Even with today's technology, the exact reason or cause of low back problems can be found in very few people. Most times, the symptoms are blamed on poor muscle tone in the back, muscle tension or spasm, back sprains, ligament or muscle tears, joint problems. Sometimes nerves from the spinal cord can be irritated by slipped discs causing buttock or leg pain. This may also cause numbness, tingling, or weakness in the legs.

People who are in poor physical condition or do work that includes heavy labor or long periods of sitting or standing are at greater risk for low back problems. These people also get better more slowly. Emotional stress or long periods of inactivity may make back symptoms seem worse.

Low back problems are often painful. But the good news is that very few people turn out to have a major problem with the bones or joints of the back or a dangerous medical condition.

Things To Do About Low Back Problems

Seeing a health care provider

Many people who develop mild low back discomfort may not need to see a health care provider right away. Often, within a few days, the symptoms go away without any treatment.

A visit to your health care provider is a good idea if:

- Your symptoms are severe.
- The pain is keeping you from doing things that you do every day.
- The problem does not go away within a few days.

If you also have problems controlling your bowel or bladder, if you feel numb in the groin or rectal area, or if there is extreme leg weakness, call your health care provider right away.

Your health care provider will check to see if you have a medical illness causing your back problem (chances are you will not). Your health care provider can also help you get some relief from your symptoms.

Your health care provider will:

- Ask about your symptoms and what they keep you from doing.
- Ask about your medical history.
- Give you a physical exam.

Talking About Your Symptoms

Your health care provider will want to know about your back problem. Here are some examples of the kinds of questions he or she may ask you. You can write down the answers in the space below each question:

When did your back symptoms start?

Which of your daily activities are you not able to do because of your back symptoms?

Is there anything you do that makes the symptoms better or worse?

Have you noticed any problem with your legs?

Around the time your symptoms began, did you have a fever or symptoms of pain or burning when urinating?

Talking About Your Medical History

Be sure to tell your health care provider about your general health and about illnesses you have had in the past. Here are some questions your health care provider may ask you about your medical history. You can write your answers in the space below each question:

Have you had a problem with your back in the past? If so, when?

____

____

____

What medical illnesses have you had (for example, cancer, arthritis, or diseases of the immune system)?

____

____

____

Which medicines do you take regularly?

____

____

____

Have you ever used intravenous (IV) drugs?

____

____

____

Have you recently lost weight without trying?

____

____

You should also tell your health care provider about anything you may be doing for your symptoms: medicines you are taking, creams or ointments you are using, and other home remedies.

Having A Physical Exam

Your health care provider will examine your back. Even after a careful physical examination, it may not be possible for your health care provider to tell you the exact cause of your low back problem. But you most likely will find out that your symptoms are not being caused by a dangerous medical condition. Very few people (about 1 in 200) have low back symptoms caused by such conditions. You probably wont need special tests (page 11) if you have had low back symptoms for only a few weeks.

Getting Relief

Your health care provider will help you get relief from your pain, discomfort, or other symptoms. A number of medicines and other treatments help with low back symptoms. The good news is that most people start feeling better soon.

Proven Treatments

Medicine often helps relieve low back symptoms. The type of medicine that your health care provider recommends depends on your symptoms and how uncomfortable you are.

- If your symptoms are mild to moderate, you may get the relief you need from an over-the-counter (nonprescription) medicine such as acetaminophen, aspirin, or ibuprofen. These medicines usually have fewer side effects than prescription medicines and are less expensive.
- If your symptoms are severe, your health care provider may recommend a prescription medicine.
- For most people, medicine works well to control pain and discomfort. But any medicine can have side effects. For example, some people cannot take aspirin or ibuprofen because it can cause stomach irritation and even ulcers. Many medicines prescribed for low back pain can make people feel drowsy. These medicines should not be taken if you need to drive or use heavy equipment. Talk to your health care provider about the benefits and risks of any medicine recommended. If you develop side effects (such as

nausea, vomiting, rash, dizziness), stop taking the medicine, and tell your health care provider right away.

- Your health care provider may recommend one or more of the following to be used alone or along with medicine to help relieve your symptoms
- Heat or cold applied to the back. Within the first 48 hours after your back symptoms start, you may want to apply a cold pack (or a bag of ice) to the painful area for 5 to 10 minutes at a time. If your symptoms last longer than 48 hours, you may find that a heating pad or hot shower or bath helps relieve your symptoms.
- Spinal manipulation. This treatment (using the hands to apply force to the back to adjust the spine) can be helpful for some people in the first month of low back symptoms. It should only be done by a professional with experience in manipulation. You should go back to your health care provider if your symptoms have not responded to spinal manipulation within 4 weeks.

Keep in mind that everyone is different. You will have to find what works best to relieve your own back symptoms.

Other Treatments

A number of other treatments are sometimes used for low back symptoms. While these treatments may give relief for a short time, none have been found to speed recovery or keep acute back problems from returning. They may also be expensive. Such treatments include:

- Traction.
- TENS (transcutaneous electrical nerve stimulation).
- Massage.
- Biofeedback.
- Acupuncture.

- Injections into the back.
- Back corsets.
- Ultrasound.

Physical Activity

Your health care provider will want to know about the physical demands of your life (your job or daily activities). Until you feel better, your health care provider may need to recommend some changes in your activities. You will want to talk to your health care provider about your own personal situation. In general, when pain is severe, you should avoid:

- Heavy lifting.
- Lifting when twisting, bending forward, and reaching.
- Sitting for long periods of time.

The most important goal is for you to return to your normal activities as soon as it is safe. Your health care provider and (if you work) your employer can help you decide how much you are able to do safely at work. Your schedule can be gradually increased as your back improves.

Bed Rest

If your symptoms are severe, your health care provider may recommend a short period of bed rest. However, bed rest should be limited to 2 or 3 days. Lying down for longer periods may weaken muscles and bones and actually slow your recovery. If you feel that you must lie down, be sure to get up every few hours and walk around even if it hurts. Feeling a little discomfort as you return to normal activity is common and does not mean that you are hurting yourself.

About Work and Family

Back problems take time to get better. If your job or your normal daily activities make your back pain worse, it is important to communicate this to your family, supervisor, and coworkers. Put your energy into doing those things at work and at home that you are able to do comfortably. Be productive, but be clear about those tasks that you are not able to do.

Things You Can Do Now

While waiting for your back to improve, you may be able to make yourself more comfortable if you:

- Wear comfortable, low-heeled shoes.
- Make sure your work surface is at a comfortable height for you.
- Use a chair with a good lower back support that may recline slightly.
- If you must sit for long periods of time, try resting your feet on the floor or on a low stool, whichever is more comfortable.
- If you must stand for long periods of time, try resting one foot on a low stool.
- If you must drive long distances, try using a pillow or rolled-up towel behind the small of your back. Also, be sure to stop often and walk around for a few minutes.

If you have trouble sleeping, try sleeping on your back with a pillow under your knees, or sleep on your side with your knees bent and a pillow between your knees.

Exercise

A gradual return to normal activities, including exercise, is recommended. Exercise is important to your overall health and can help you to lose body fat (if needed). Even if you have mild to moderate low back symptoms, the following things can be done without putting much stress on your back:

- Walking short distances.
- Using a stationary bicycle.
- Swimming.

It is important to start any exercise program slowly and to gradually build up the speed and length of time that you do the exercise. At first, you may find that your symptoms get a little worse when you exercise or become more active. Usually, this is nothing to worry about. However, if your pain becomes severe, contact your health care provider. Once you are able to return to normal activities comfortably, your health care provider may recommend further aerobic and back exercises.

If You Are Not Getting Better

Most low back problems get better quickly, and usually within 4 weeks. If your symptoms are not getting better within this time period, you should contact your health care provider.

Special Tests

Your health care provider will examine your back again and may talk to you about getting some special tests. These may include x-rays, blood tests, or other special studies such as an MRI (magnetic resonance imaging) or CT (computerized tomography) scan of your back. These tests may help your health care provider understand why you are not getting better. Your health care provider may also want to refer you to a specialist.

Certain things, such as stress (extra pressure at home or work), personal or emotional problems, depression, or a problem with drug or alcohol use can slow recovery or make back symptoms seem worse. If you have any of these problems, tell your health care provider.

About Surgery

Even having a lot of back pain does not by itself mean you need surgery. Surgery has been found to be helpful in only 1 in 100 cases of low back problems. In some people, surgery can even cause more problems. This is especially true if your only symptom is back pain.

People with certain nerve problems or conditions such as fractures or dislocations have the best chance of being helped by surgery. In most cases, however, decisions about surgery do not have to be made right away. Most back surgery can wait for several weeks without making the condition worse.

If your health care provider recommends surgery, be sure to ask about the reason for the surgery and about the risks and benefits you might expect. You may also want to get a second opinion.

Prevention of Low Back Problems

The best way to prevent low back problems is to stay fit. If you must lift something, even after your back seems better, be sure to:

- Keep all lifted objects close to your body.
- Avoid lifting while twisting, bending forward, and reaching.

You should continue to exercise even after your back symptoms have gone away. There are many exercises that can be done to condition muscles of your body and back. You should talk to your health care provider about the exercises that would be best for you.

When Low Back Symptoms Return

More than half of the people who recover from a first episode of acute low back symptoms will have another episode within a few years. Unless your back symptoms are very different from the first episode, or you have a new medical condition, you can expect to recover quickly and fully from each episode.

While Your Back is Getting Better

It is important to remember that even though you are having a problem with your back now, most likely it will begin to feel better soon. It is important to keep in mind that you are the most important person in taking care of your back and in helping to get back to your regular activities. It may also help you to remember that:

- Most low back problems last for a short amount of time and the symptoms usually get better with little or no medical treatment.
- Low back problems can be painful. But pain rarely means that there is serious damage to your back.

- Exercise can help you to feel better faster and prevent more back problems. A regular exercise program adds to your general health and may help you get back to the things you enjoy doing.

For Further Information

The information in this booklet was based on the *Clinical Practice Guideline, Acute Low Back Problems in Adults.* The *Guideline* was developed by a non-Federal panel of experts sponsored by the Agency for Health Care Policy and Research. Other guidelines on common health problems are available, and more are being developed.

For more information about guidelines or to receive a free copy of *Understanding Acute Low Back Problems*, call toll-free 800-358-9295, or write to:

Agency for Health Care Policy and Research
Publications Clearinghouse
P.O. Box 8547
Silver Spring, MD 20907

U.S. Department of Health and Human Services
Public Health Service
Agency for Health Care Policy and Research
Executive Office Center, Suite 501
2101 East Jefferson Street Rockville, MD 20852

AHCPR Publication No. 95-0644; December 1994

What you have just finished reading is the BEST EVIDENCE we currently have to give you about acute back pain.

Other recommendations should be scrutinized very closely.

Chapter 10

My Opinion Is The Only One That Counts And Other Ironies of Alternative Medicine

All I have learned of any value has been self-taught.

—Charles Darwin

It is a matter of "My Opinion is the Only One That Counts" because opinion, belief, and intuition form the core of alternative medicine. It became increasingly clear to me that the way chiropractic worked is that once you become indoctrinated about one technique, you dismiss any other method of treatment.

One practitioner will believe passionately that ice massage and bed rest are the cures for low back pain. Another will argue just as vocally that electrical muscle stimulation is the way to go. Still another will insist that spinal manipulation is the best solution. If they believe in a newer or not as widely used technique, it may be because they have recently attended a seminar where that technique has been taught. It is not uncommon for a chiropractor to go to a seminar and then diagnose every patient who comes into the office the next day with the problem that can "best" be remedied by the new technique. It is not science they are looking to after all. It is akin to adolescent experimentation.

There is simply no independent thought inside the chiropractic cave. A chiropractor and management consultant once said to me with a straight face, "I am truly convinced that the vertebral subluxation is the number one cause of disease in the world today. I also am a firm believer that chiropractic is the answer to *this* world's health problems." Is there also another world that he hopes to conquer someday? If you are not shaking your head or laughing over his comments, then you have missed the point of this book.

In chiropractic, so much brainwashing takes place, so much of a cult mentality is encouraged, so much faulty reasoning is reinforced that even among chiropractors who claim to reject most principles of the profession there is still a fundamental attachment to non-evidence-based approaches. It is similar to an addiction.

Even years after you quit smoking you may crave cigarettes. Likewise, even after renouncing the theosophy of chiropractic, a practitioner may find himself or herself touting treatments that have no clinical foundation.

I was one of them for a long time. I suspected most of the techniques used by chiropractors were unscientific but I continued to count them among the treatments that I offered my patients because they seem so satisfied with them. My favorites and theirs included electrical muscle stimulation, ultrasound, traction, moist heat, massage and ice massage as well as spinal manipulation for pain other than in the low back.

In the preface to this book Dale Dauten raved about my use of an electrical muscle stimulator to treat his back pain. That was in 1995 and I had yet to be convinced that this approach was useless because so many of my patients responded positively to it. Dale still insists it felt great.

Ah, the allure of the placebo – for both patient and practitioner. Even though I sensed from my first day in chiropractic school that this "science" was questionable, I was not ready to fully acknowledge my suspicion until eleven years or so after graduation.

I was helped along in this "epiphany" by stepping outside the intellectual and academic boundaries (and I use the term loosely) imposed by the chiropractic profession on itself. In the late 1980s I started reading books, articles, and studies not endorsed – in fact, shunned – by chiropractic schools and practicing chiropractors.

In the mid-1990s I hopped on the cyber highway and found pages and pages and more pages of information challenging chiropractic theosophy. The Internet showed me how little I knew and led me to conclude that the average patient and the average chiropractor were totally clueless. After all, chiropractors at that time were the only professionals licensed in Arizona not required to fulfill a continuing education requirement. Today they are required to complete just twelve hours of continuing ed each year. By contrast, I completed more than

198 hours of continuing education programs in 1998 alone. My continuing education classes focused primarily on forensics (based on scientific fact) and allowed me to stay current in my roles as a certified fraud examiner, certified disability examiner, and peer reviewer. The more I study the more I realize that the educational process is never-ending -- a view that contradicts the most sacred principles of chiropractic.

By 1996, I understood what my role needed to be as a practitioner. The word "physician" is Greek for "teacher" and I realized that what I tell people is far more important than what I do for them. I gradually gave up performing all therapies except spinal manipulation for acute low back pain. I say "gradually" because my patients so enjoyed the hot packs, the ultrasound, and the electrical muscle stimulation that it was difficult for me to let go of these placebos that people so firmly believed were helping them. But I knew that if I were going to pursue evidence-based care of back pain I had to relinquish the unproven remedies.

Now my awakening to the truth has come full circle. I am getting a Ph.D. in health services, focusing on scientifically valid ways to combat back pain.

The Opposite Viewpoint

> *To argue with a man who has renounced his reason is like giving medicine to the dead.*
>
> —Thomas Paine

When a professional organization representing a particular health care discipline invests the time and energy necessary to create a uniform standard of care, that document should contain some very basic elements (such as a template to help a practitioner determine the appropriate number of visits for a patient's particular ailment) and should be richly annotated with references to clinical studies. That is not what you would find in the latest International Chiropractors Association's (ICA) *Recommended Clinical Protocols and Guidelines for the Practice of Chiropractic.*

What you will find is a recommendation for "applicable procedures" during initial visits, such as x-rays. *Remember that evidence-based medicine says patients should not undergo x-rays for mechanical back pain within the first four weeks of the onset of pain.* You will also find a recommendation for maintenance care after the patient's condition has been treated, but as we noted in Chapter 8, there is no evidence that maintenance care is necessary or helpful.

You would find that the definition of "acute" (as opposed to chronic) pain is "a new condition, not exceeding 12 months [sic] duration." Twelve months? Evidence-based medicine says 80 percent of mechanical back pain lasts no more than six weeks. But by suggesting that acute pain routinely lasts a year the Guidelines underscore a bias toward excessive treatment.

The document even delineates phases of care when a "subluxation" is found on an x-ray. Initial care should last from fourteen to forty-five days after the first visit; "reconstruction" care (what is that?) should occur between forty-five and 180 days after first visit; "supportive" (that is, maintenance) care should be provided "as necessitated by subjective and/or objective findings and documentation." That translates to "as determined by how greedy the chiropractor is willing to be." And again, remember: the existence of subluxations has never been proven.

The Guidelines also say "the rationale for chiropractic management in chronic pain dysfunction syndromes of particular origin is well-established in the scientific literature." Where is the information about the specific studies? Nowhere in the document you will be shocked to learn. If you are going to mention scientific literature, then you should be able to cite specific clinical studies to support your claims. In these Guidelines evidence does not even make an appearance.

The document makes two other pronouncements that I find especially interesting. One is "...chiropractic care should begin at birth when subluxations are likely to occur ... Given the chiropractor's objective and the overwhelming supportive evidence mentioned above, chiropractic care can begin shortly after birth and be followed by a lifetime of continuing care" [what I like to call "from the womb to the tomb"]. I find it intriguing that the language is "given the chiropractor's objective..." What exactly is the chiropractor's objective? To help the patient get better at a reasonable cost or to create a lifelong dependency that will benefit only the practitioner? Because it is so suspect the "chiropractor's objective" should never determine whether or not the patient undergoes a lifetime of treatments.

Remember what we said about pediatric chiropractic care? It is rarely if ever necessary or recommended. Yet here is the International Chiropractors Association saying without hesitation or exception (or any citations for this "overwhelming supportive evidence") that your newborn should see a chiro. I like to refer to this as "womb to tomb" chiropractic care! That is not an original phrase, yet it is perfect for the occasion.

The other pronouncement is just laughable. Here it is: "The necessity of long-term palliative or supportive [read "maintenance"] care should accomplish one or more of the following goals in order to be considered necessary and appropriate: [these are randomly selected from a list of 10 goals: 1) increase stamina, endurance and activity tolerance; 2) improve mental attitude; 3) to attain optimal expression of life."

I hardly know where to begin commenting on this. First of all, it is written so poorly that it is almost incomprehensible. "The necessity ... should accomplish ... the following goals ... to be considered necessary and appropriate"? Secondly, what is "optimal expression of life"? Is that different from quality of life, and if so, how? Third, are not there about 4,000 other options for "improving mental attitude" and increasing "stamina, endurance and activity tolerance" that do not require you to invest tens of thousands of dollars and remain beholden to a chiropractor for the rest of your life? Think about it: is there any other health care profession anywhere that recommends a lifetime of ongoing care? If your medical doctor, dentist, physical therapist, or optometrist said, "I want you to come and see me once a month for the rest of your life," you would be surprised to say the least. Why are we not just as skeptical when a chiropractor suggests that much care?

The Guidelines go on to invoke "research" to artificially boost chiropractic's credibility. "The current body of research in this area supports the observation that initial degenerative changes are measurable within one week of the occurrence of vertebral subluxation and other malpositioned articulations and structures." In English, what does this mean? And where is the research they are talking about?

The document goes on to say that weekly or semi-monthly office visits are appropriate. "When interference to the nervous system is reduced, the body's capacity to heal and thrive is rekindled," the Guidelines say. "It is imperative that chiropractic care should begin as soon as possible. Chiropractic care should continue in accordance with the patient's needs and the chiropractor's clinical opinion for the life of the patient." These are the messages being conveyed by a professional organization to its members and potential members. The document is devoid of science, logic, evidence or, in most places, simple common sense. You can read the entire document for yourself by going online to www.chiropractic.org

and then clicking on "Guidelines." These quotes are taken from Chapter 11.

It is becoming increasingly difficult to strip chiropractic away from the "mantle" of legitimacy bestowed on it not only by documents such as these Guidelines (that couch a belief system in scientific-sounding words) but also by expanding government acceptance of its tenets. Not long ago the U.S. Congress considered a bill called The Chiropractic Patients' Freedom of Choice Act of 2001, which provides "reimbursement under the Medicare program for all physicians' services furnished by doctors of chiropractic within the scope of their license." At the time of this writing, the bill (identified as H.R. 902) had not passed. But here we have the legislative branch of the United States government mulling over a proposal essentially to write a blank check to the chiropractic community bearing the signature of American taxpayers. At least 24 members of Congress want you to pay for everything a chiropractor might do for patients 65 and over. That may or may not include acupuncture, electrical muscle stimulation, etc, etc. Might it also include pubic hair analysis?

> ***The Medicare system already is teetering on the brink of insolvency and our inspired, visionary lawmakers want to put even more financial pressure on the system by forcing the executive branch of the government to pay for pseudo-medicine.***

If your mother or husband or sister had a chronic illness (such as Parkinson's disease or diabetes) would you rather that a chiropractic adjustment be paid for by Medicare or that badly needed medications were paid for? I can almost guarantee you that Medicare will not cover both. And if the chiropractic community gets its way a prescription drug plan likely would fly out the window. Are you happy at the prospect of your tax dollars paying for tens of thousands of monthly chiropractic adjustments that are in all likelihood completely unnecessary and may eclipse a prescription drug plan? And are you happy that this bill could open the floodgates to all kinds of alternative treatments becoming acceptable to Medicare?

Chiropractic has been called the "legislated profession" because so much of its acceptance and expansion into the health insurance arena is linked to a long-standing, massive, intensive lobbying effort on the part of chiropractors and chiropractic organizations, not to mentioned their core of believers.

> ***As you have learned, chiropractors rely on anecdotes to recruit more patients into their practice. Chiropractic uses that same approach when dealing with state and federal legislators by providing patients who tout their "success" stories to give credence to the necessity of mandating coverage.***

Since my real education began I have discovered that most people who see chiropractors on a regular basis typically fall into one of three groups: 1) they had an injury or pain initially and continue to trust their chiropractors; 2) they have a "world owes me" mentality where their auto accident or work injury is the perfect excuse for them to complain of pain forever and leave behind their work life; or 3) they are committing fraud. (Health care fraud is a topic for another book that I am currently considering.)

The next time you are considering which health professional to go to, think about who is a bona fide scientific practitioner versus who has had their training through indoctrination. Think about which practitioner is dedicated to helping people and which one has recently expanded his or her practice simply to improve their own financial bottom line.

The Myth of Whiplash

> *It is better to be a mouse in a cat's mouth than a man in a lawyer's hands.*
>
> –Spanish proverb

Whiplash is defined as an injury to your neck. Treating whiplash is one of the staples of many chiropractic offices; they depend on you and your neighbors to get in car accidents and hurt your neck. News flash: we have no evidence-based research that spinal manipulation can do anything for whiplash. Remember that manipulation is not indicated in the neck area. We know that as a result of manipulation of your neck, you can suffer a stroke and die, or become paralyzed or endure "other malpositioned articulations and structures" to use the ridiculous terminology from the ICA Guidelines.

✔ Whether whiplash is even real depends on what you read. A study in Germany found that in a group of people with neck pain following an injury, all of them were better by six weeks after the injury, whether they underwent treatment or did nothing. What have I been harping on for nine chapters? That the vast majority of patients with back or neck pain get better within six weeks regardless of what treatment they undergo. In the vast majority of whiplash claimants, radiological findings are not helpful in demonstrating the existence of a whiplash, because the injury is typically to soft tissue that does not show up on an x-ray. We have already talked about the foolishness of exposing yourself to unnecessary ionizing radiation.

> ***In most whiplash claimants the injury is nothing more than a minor soft tissue strain with temporary symptoms. Instead of encouraging patients to worry themselves unnecessarily by insisting on lots and lots of treatment, practitioners should be reassuring patients that their injury will most likely resolve within days or weeks at most with minimal or no intervention.***

Psychological distress can actually make pain seem worse. To ease people out of their fear practitioners need to let them know immediately that they will be okay. In the case of whiplash, measuring the success of treatment is accomplished as much by observing the behavior of the patient as by determining whether the injury has healed. With whiplash (and back pain in general) it does not matter what we do. It is a self-limiting condition.

But try convincing chiropractors of that. In a large metropolitan area you are likely to see more than 25,000 motor vehicle accidents every year. We know that as many as half of all people injured in an auto accident will seek medical care for their injuries, and the majority of that care will be provided by chiropractors. Some chiropractic offices specialize in treating auto accident injuries and they advertise in as many places as they can to get the word out -- on billboards, in the yellow pages of the phone book and on fliers dropped off at thousands of homeowners' front doors. They may team up with one or more of hundreds of personal injury (PI) lawyers that advertise in the yellow pages in any large metropolitan area. The grayness and unsubstantiated nature of subluxation -- and even whiplash -- lend themselves perfectly to a PI lawyer's perspective. After all, what do attorneys do? They argue the gray zones. I am confident that these words will be read to me again during future court proceedings as personal injury lawyers try to muddy the waters in the minds of jurors.

Chiropractors and personal injury lawyers make a perfect marriage. I ask you not to be the minister who marries them. Here is what may happen if you go to a personal injury lawyer first after an auto accident: he or she will discuss your case and then refer you to a chiropractor. You will get care you do not need and the insurance company will be hit with the bill as part of a lawsuit. If you go to a chiropractor first, he or she may refer you to an attorney. Either way, by the time the case settles, you are going to be left with less money than the lawyer and the chiropractor both take away. Personal injury case law rewards pain and suffering instead of health and recovery. There is no money on the horizon for the chiro or the lawyer if you return to a healthy state quickly. That is why lawyer-induced disability is running rampant in our country.

If you decide to contact an attorney after your car accident, do so in the same spirit and skeptical fashion as you would choose a chiropractor.

Science and Truth vs. Quackery and Greed

> *Most of the people teaching evidence-based medicine in a variety of settings have encountered at least on occasion reactions of, at best, skepticism, and at worst, hostility.*
>
> --Roman Z. Jaeschke

Because I have successfully challenged chiropractic theosophy on many occasions, I have personally experienced numerous obstacles to being an evidence-based practitioner. These have run the gamut from pure ignorance ("No, I have never heard of evidence-based care") to hostility (complaints filed against me with the state Board of Chiropractic Examiners) to felonious activity (a brick thrown at my office window and a death threat left on my voice mail). I have friends throughout North America who have been practicing chiropractors and now embrace evidence-based medicine, and they too have experienced similar obstacles.

What I find interesting is that we are not opposed by legitimate practitioners, be they M.D.s or evidence-based chiropractors. It is only the people who feel threatened by truth who go out of their way to discredit evidence-based medicine (EBM). Why would they be threatened by the definition of evidence-based medicine?

EBM Defined

EBM is "evidence-based medicine" ~ simply the conscientious and judicious use of current best evidence from clinical care research in the management of individual patients. EBM, with its emphasis on ethics and accuracy, jeopardizes chiropractors' very livelihoods and the chiropractors find ways to fight against the truth.

✔ In North America, an evidence-based practitioner faced a board complaint filed against him by twelve chiropractors whose offices were near his. They objected to his peer reviews and independent medical exams (IMEs), saying they were biased and unfair. The matter took several years to resolve and in the meantime the evidence-based practitioner had to put his building up for sale because the complaint had affected his livelihood. Within 24 hours after the building was placed on the market the issue before the board was resolved in his favor.

✔ An evidence-based practitioner in the Midwest was persecuted by other chiropractors to the point of being forced to give up his entire peer review/independent medical exam practice.

✔ In the Southwest an evidence-based practitioner received so many death threats that he had to get the police involved and now carries a weapon with him wherever he goes.

If they cannot stop you through intimidation, chiropractors and their backers will try to get legislation passed at the state level that restricts a consultant's free trade. Some bills limit a chiropractor's consulting work (peer reviews, independent medical exams) to just five percent of the practitioner's total income.

✔ The legislation would restrict exposing chiropractors like the one we mentioned in Chapter 1, who treated a man with low back pain 202 times! Not only was this beyond excessive, she did not even treat his low back. For the first 101 treatments she shoved the top bone in his neck to the right. During the next 101 visits she moved his atlas to the left. He was never examined and never received the treatment that would have been appropriate for him, which was a short course of spinal manipulation of the low back. I performed a peer review of her documents at the request of the patient's health insurance carrier. I determined that the care she provided had been excessive and inappropriate. I said this patient could have been treated appropriately through evidence-based medicine. What do you think happened?

The insurance company denied the claim and a complaint was brought against me by the chiropractor. I defended my report before the Board of Chiropractic Examiners and I was exonerated.

Thoughts on Evidence-Based Medicine

Evidence-based medicine within the alternative medicine community (and particularly chiropractic) will never succeed unless and until the general public and patients develop an understanding of what evidence-based health care is. That is the purposes of this book: to disseminate knowledge to you the consumer, providing you with the knowledge to make intelligent choices. I don't think an alternative health care provider is willingly going to embrace evidence-based medicine because it is financially unrewarding to do so. As Plato said, "In general, dishonesty is always more profitable than honesty."

If evidence-based medicine is to grow in popularity, consumers have to demand change. With the limitless access that we have to medical information, it is we – the U.S. patient base – who need to be the motivating force for change. As patients we need to understand and accept that sometimes it is in our best interests to decline care even when it is available for "free." It could end up harming you even if it does not cost anything.

Think about how conventional medicine has evolved. Think about how dramatically the technology has changed in just the past decade, let alone the past fifty years. In the 1960s, for example, heart bypass surgery was not an option for patients. Today it saves hundreds of thousands of lives every year. As William J. Mayo said in 1928, "The glory of medicine is that it is constantly moving forward, that there's always more to learn."

Now, think about chiropractic care. D.D. Palmer introduced it to the world in 1895. He claimed that a man's hearing was restored when his thoracic (middle) spine was manipulated. That was the beginning of the chiropractic profession. Today, more than a hundred and five years later, the techniques have not changed substantially. People in Iowa at the turn of the last century might have believed that chiropractic was a miracle or was just the treatment they needed to cure their ills, but does it make sense to adopt the identical belief in the 21st century?

As we have shown, chiropractic is not a risk-free panacea. You and your family deserve safe and therapeutic treatments based on scientific investigation and proof,

and not based on provider opinion and case histories or miraculous stories.

Start doing your own investigation. Evaluate your treatment options, understand the risks and if you have not already, interview your provider about his or her background, philosophy, and experience. Do not feel intimidated or defensive. Then make an intelligent choice about the best care for you.

This book is intended to be the first step in your journey of self-education. It is a walk composed of thousands of steps, not overnight discovery. People will only have power over you if you give it to them.

Do not give your "health power" to any provider, especially a chiropractor.

Chapter 11

My Future For Chiropractic

We know that, if chiropractic is to thrive, numerous changes need to be made. Oh, it *could* continue to survive without change like it has for the past 106+ years, the unwanted step-child of the medical profession. The same ineffective practices will continue. In this stagnant industry chiropractic schools churn out "grads" with no where to go, desperate for clients they are not truly equipped to help but from whom they can certainly take advantage.

If we had free reign to make changes, what changes should we make?

My daughter likes to play a computer fantasy game called "Sims." For those of you who are not familiar with Sims ~ short for "simulation" ~ it is a game where you create your own world, build your own homes and cities, airport networks, amusement parks, and even control the characters. What I am presenting here is a "Sims" version of the future of chiropractic. So join me, King Chiropractor, and we will make the world a better place.

The Education

We would start at the beginning by increasing the entrance requirements for chiropractic college. We would make it a mandatory requirement that all future doctors of chiropractic would hold a bachelor's degree in Biology or some other similar scientific pursuit ~ anatomy, chemistry. It would be the same for all colleges: a four-year degree with a grade point average of 2.5 or higher. No longer would an application be accepted solely based on the fact it was signed by a warm body. By increasing the entrance requirements we would also increase the quality of students. I am sure you agree: this is a necessary first step.

Next, we would limit the number of chiropractors teaching future chiropractors in the colleges, especially chiropractors that have been taught by other chiropractors who do not have a bachelor's degree in the subject they are teaching. Anatomy and chemistry should be taught by anatomists and chemists, not chiropractors. To have a chiropractor without a bachelor's degree, teaching other chiropractors in the same institution that they graduated from, is not in the best interests of anyone.

The new chiropractic colleges need to acquire the federal dollars to hire and perform sound scientific research. These researchers should not be chiropractors researching philosophical anecdotes, but scholars researching medicine using sound methodological principles. These researchers would have no chiropractic background or biases. They would be data doctors, bona fide research scientists.

After the entrance requirements are increased and quality of instructors improved, we would then alter the curriculum. We would start by deleting all the philosophical classes from the curriculum. Chiropractic is a physical science, not mental, not a religion, not some new science-of-the-week. If it is not evidence-based, it is not in the curriculum.

Technique classes would all but be deleted. It does not take a lot of skill to manipulate or crack someone's back. The true skill comes in knowing when to treat and when not to treat.

Another vital change is in the area of patients for chiropractic students. Currently students treat other students and their friends or family members. To be called a "doctor" you should actually see, diagnose, and treat sick people. In my clinical days stories abounded of students hiring prostitutes to come in as patients to perform breast exams on. This last sentence gives a succinct picture of the flaws in the professional education. Chiropractors doing breast exams ~ that is more than a little outrageous, First of all, breast exams should not be in our scope of practice. One way to provide chiropractic students with actual sick patients is to secure rotations at local hospitals or outpatient facilities. By providing these new chiropractic interns real patients, they could become actual members of the health care community. Learning on real patients and becoming actual members of the health care community are absolute musts in the fantasy "Sims" world of chiropractic.

Another major improvement would be to include pharmacology education as part of all chiropractors' curriculum. Are we nuts, giving drugs to chiropractors, prescription pads to abuse? Answer: yes. Remember: by the time this would occur in the new chiropractic fantasyland prior changes would have already taken place. A bachelor's degree with a minimum grade point average, pharmacists, anatomists, and chemists teaching those classes, and only evidence-based spinal manipulation being taught. Many things would have occurred before we put the prescription pad in the hands of the new "Sims" chiropractor. This privilege of being able to write prescriptions would also be limited to only a few drug classes. It would be restricted to lower-level painkillers, anti-inflammatories, and a small group of antibiotics. Most patients in the acute phase could benefit from at least one of these medication types.

The point of all these recommendations is to bring future chiropractors up to the standards of the medical community.

Summarizing, the college aspect of my future for chiropractic is:

- Improve the entrance the requirements to chiropractic colleges, requiring a four-year degree, and a minimum grade point average.
- Improve the teaching staff by limiting the number of chiropractors teaching chiropractors.
- Remove the philosophical belief systems. Replace it with true evidence-based medical science.
- Secure the money to fund solid methodological research, performed by actual researchers.
- Add pharmacology to the curriculum.
- Secure rotations in hospitals or outpatient facilities.

All of these requirements are important in the new-world chiropractic realm. My personal opinion is that the most vital change is securing the funds to do the necessary research supporting, one way or the other, the benefits of spinal manipulation.

Paradigm Shift

If research supports any benefit currently to spinal manipulative therapy, it is for acute low back pain in adults only. This would be the launching pad ~ the initial starting point for future research and for the new chiropractic profession. From this starting point, new doctors, the colleges, and medical researchers could undertake the task of scientific discovery. Through sound methodological clinical trials, the question can be answered: is there is any benefit to spinal manipulation?

Based on this new research, clinical practice algorithms, or "guidelines" would be established with strict research protocols for possible new treatments for pain and injury to body areas other than the lower back. Presently there are guidelines and algorithms for acute low back pain in adults, only.

Many of the criticisms of chiropractic would disappear if the profession embraced the evidence-based movement. The unscientific cult stigma could be replaced by a solid evidence-based and honorable position within the scientific community of chiropractic. Evidence-based medicine would greatly decrease the almost endless practice variations seen within the chiropractic community.

There are over 400 chiropractic techniques in existence. Of these, little, if any, research supports their use for the treatment of anything. The consistent use of evidence-based medicine methods for diagnosis, special testing, and treatment would enhance chiropractic standing in the medical and consumer communities. In the scientific community this would also provide the current, most up-to-date information for the treatment of acute low back pain. The graduating chiropractors would be evidence-based practitioners of spinal manipulation. As research determines what techniques are worthwhile and which are not, only the evidence-based techniques would be offered in the chiropractic curriculum. Once they graduated, practitioners would not need to resort to unsubstantiated techniques in their clinical practice.

In our perfect world the chiropractic profession must get away from any sort of religious philosophy, particularly in regard to what it detects and treats. Doctors can be religious, a science cannot.

Self-Imposed Regulation

From a treatment standpoint, presently the evidence only mildly supports spinal manipulation for acute low back pain in adults. This is it for now. Chiropractors have been saying that will change but it has not ~ for decades. For the immediate future the chiropractic profession would limit care to consumers with lower back pain. Chiropractors would treat only adults between eighteen and fifty-five who have acute, mechanical low back pain. They would not treat nerve root pain or serious pathologies. This means no kids, no pets, no mid-backs, no necks. Of truly great interest would be the financially devastating effect this would have on whiplash cases. The numbers vary, but figures show that chiropractors make over 85% of all their income from whiplash. The remainder is maintenance types of care. The rest is too insignificant to be of importance. As the new colleges produce research to show the benefits, if any, to treating the mid-back or the neck, these practices could expand, bringing true benefits to the injured.

> ***A final observation: chiropractors would be similar in scope of practice and in community respect as dentists and podiatrists. The new chiropractor would be a "portal of entry provider" offering a standard of care to maintain. They would have limited prescription rights. They would have a clearly-defined scope of practice.***

By incorporating these basic suggestions, I do not believe there are currently enough licensed chiropractors in the United States to handle the amount of patients that would be made available to them. Remember: approximately 85% of the population, at any given time, will have severe enough acute low back pain to limit their ability to work. Right now the numbers indicate that chiropractors treat between 3-7% of the population, and these people tend to be those who will believe anything. When the public trusts chiropractors, then they will allow chiropractors to treat them.

The bottom line, as we should see it, is that the public has not bought into the chiropractic philosophy to any degree for over 106 years. Without new direction, based on evidence, I do not believe that chiropractic will continue for much longer. It might be able to survive to a small degree but it will not continue in any important way, shape, or form, and only as they function now.

There are signs of chiropractic's lack of inclusion being seen around the world. Currently in British Columbia, Canada, they will not pay for most chiropractic treatments. Quebec has never covered chiropractic services. Newfoundland will no longer cover chiropractic care. According to the World Health Organization, France is the number one country in the world for providing health care. As I understand it chiropractic is illegal in that country. There are more chiropractors in the United States than any other country. That does not say much good about us does it? We rank 37th in the international health community.

If the chiropractic industry swings back to honest, ethical, evidence-based practices, it is a win-win situation. The chiropractic community would finally achieve the level of acceptance and respect it has so desperately sought since its creation back in 1895. Chiropractors win, third parties win, consumers win. **Do you think it will happen**? *Never!* The reason? Chiropractic is the ultimate definition of insanity. By insanity I mean doing the same thing over and over again and expecting a different result. I suspect 106 years from now chiropractors will still be treating subluxations ~ subluxations that do not exist on people who do not have them. Chiropractors will still be practicing in strip malls, no different than they do today. People will be hurt. Insanity!

Appendix A

Useful Resources

Acute Low Back Problems in Adults: Assessment and Treatment

Quick Reference Guide Number 14
AHCPR Publication No. 95-0643: December 1994

Attention Clinicians:

The *Clinical Practice Guideline* on which this *Quick Reference Guide for Clinicians* is based was developed by a multidisciplinary, private-sector panel comprising health care professionals and a consumer representative sponsored by the Agency for Health Care Policy and Research (AHCPR).

Panel members were:

Stanley J. Bigos, MD (Chair)
G. Richard Braen, MD
Richard A. Deyo, MD, MPH
John L. Hart, DO
Robert B. Keller, MD
Matthew H. Liang, MD, MPH
Margareta Nordin, Dr. Med. Sc.
Malcolm H. Pope, Dr. Med. Sc., PhD
Donald H. Stewart, Jr., MD
John J. Triano, DC, MA
Dennis Turk, PhD
James Weinstein, DO
Reverend O. Richard Bowyer
Kathleen C. Brown, PhD, RN
Scott Haldeman, MD, PhD, DC
Ernest W. Johnson, MD
Daniel K. Kido, MD
Roger M. Nelson, PhD, PTT
Bernice D. Owen, PhD, RN
Richard K. Schwartz, MS, OTR
Jeffrey L. Susman, MD
Lucius Tripp, MD, MPH
Clark Watts, MD, JD

Special consultants to the panel were: Michele Batti, PT, PhD; Claire Bombardier, MD; Nortin Hadler, MD; Alf Nachemson, MD, PhD; Gordon Waddell, MD. John Holland, MD, MPH and John Webster, MD served as project directors. Project methodologists were David Schriger, MD, MPH and Paul Shekelle, MD,MPH.

An explicit, science-based methodology was employed along with expert clinical judgment to develop specific statements on patient assessment and management on acute low back problems. Extensive literature searches were conducted and critical reviews and syntheses were used to evaluate empirical evidence and significant outcomes. Peer review and pilot testing were undertaken to evaluate the validity, reliability, and utility of the guideline in clinical practice.

This Quick Reference Guide for Clinicians presents a clinical strategy for applying the statements and recommendations from the *Clinical Practice Guideline*. The latter provides a description of the guideline development process, thorough analysis and discussion of the available research, critical evaluation of the assumptions and knowledge of the field, more complete information for health care decision making, consideration for patients with special needs, and references. Decisions to adopt particular recommendations from either publication must be made by practitioners in light of available resources and circumstances presented by the individual patient. AHCPR invites comments and suggestions from users for consideration in development and updating of future guidelines.

Please send written comments to:

Director, Office of the Forum
for Quality and Effectiveness in Health Care
AHCPR, Willco Building, Suite 310
6000 Executive Boulevard
Rockville, MD 20852.

Abstract

This *Quick Reference Guide for Clinicians* contains highlights from the *Clinical Practice Guideline* version of Acute Low Back Problems in Adults, which was developed by a private-sector panel of health care providers and consumers. The *Quick Reference Guide* is an example of how a clinician might implement the panel's findings and recommendations on the management of acute low back problems in working-age adults. Topics covered include the initial assessment of patients presenting with acute low back problems, identification of red flags that may indicate the presence of a serious underlying medical condition, initial management, special studies and diagnostic considerations, and further management considerations. Instructions for clinical testing for sciatic tension, recommendations for sitting and unassisted lifting, tests for identification of clinical pathology, and algorithms for patient management are included.

Suggested Citation

This document is in the public domain and may be used and reprinted without special permission. AHCPR appreciates citation as to source and the suggested format is provided below: Bigos S, Bowyer O, Braen G, et al. Acute Low Back Problems in Adults. *Clinical Practice Guideline*, Quick Reference Guide Number.

14. Rockville, MD: U.S. Department of Health and Human Services, Public Health Service, Agency for Health Care Policy and Research, AHCPR Pub. No. 95-0643. December 1994.

Purpose and Scope

Low back problems affect virtually everyone at some time during their life. Surveys indicate a yearly prevalence of symptoms in 50 percent of working age adults; 15-20 percent seek medical care. Low back problems rank high among the reasons for physician office visits and are costly in terms of medical treatment, lost productivity, and non-monetary costs such as diminished ability to perform or enjoy usual activities. In fact, for persons under age 45, low back problems are the most common cause of disability.

Acute low back problems are defined as activity intolerance due to lower back or back-related leg symptoms of less than 3 months' duration. About 90 percent of patients with acute low back problems spontaneously recover activity tolerance within 1 month. The approach to a new episode in a patient with a recurrent low back problem is similar to that of a new acute episode.

The findings and recommendations included in the *Clinical Practice Guideline* define a paradigm shift away from focusing care exclusively on the pain and toward helping patients improve activity tolerance. The intent of this Quick Reference Guide is to bring to life this paradigm shift. The guide provides information on the detection of serious conditions that occasionally cause low back symptoms (conditions such as spinal fracture, tumor, infection, cauda equina syndrome, or non-spinal conditions). However, treatment of these conditions is beyond the scope of this guideline. In addition, the guideline does not address the care of patients younger than 18 years or those with chronic back problems (back-related activity limitations of greater than 3 months' duration).

Initial Assessment

- Seek potentially dangerous underlying conditions.
- In the absence of signs of dangerous conditions, there is no need for special studies since 90 percent of patients will recover spontaneously within 4 weeks.

A focused medical history and physical examination are sufficient to assess the patient with an acute or recurrent limitation due to low back symptoms of less than 4 weeks duration. Patient responses and findings on the history and physical examination, referred to as "red flags" (Table 12), raise suspicion of serious underlying spinal conditions. Their absence rules out the need for special studies during the first 4 weeks of symptoms when spontaneous recovery is expected. The medical history and physical _examination can also alert the clinician to non- spinal pathology (abdominal, pelvic, thoracic) that can present as low back symptoms. Acute low back symptoms can then be classified into one of three working categories:

- Potentially serious spinal condition: tumor, infection, spinal fracture, or a major neurologic compromise, such as cauda equina syndrome, suggested by a red flag.
- Sciatica: back-related lower limb symptoms suggesting lumbosacral nerve root compromise.
- Nonspecific back symptoms: occurring primarily in the back and suggesting neither nerve root compromise nor a serious underlying condition.

Table 1. Red Flags For Potentially Serious Conditions

❖ Medical History

In addition to detecting serious conditions and categorizing back symptoms, the medical history establishes rapport between the clinician and patient. The patient's description of present symptoms and limitations, duration of symptoms, and history of previous episodes defines the problem. It also provides insight into concerns, expectations, and nonphysical (psychological and socioeconomic) issues that may alter the patient's response to treatment. Assessment tools such as pain drawings and visual analog pain-rating scales may help further document the patient's perceptions and progress.

A patient's estimate of personal activity intolerance due to low back symptoms contributes to the clinical assessment of the severity of the back problem, guides treatment, and establishes a baseline for recommending daily activities and evaluating progress.

Open-ended questions, such as those listed below, can gauge the need for further discussion or specific inquiries for more detailed information:

- What are your symptoms?
- Pain, numbness, weakness, stiffness?
- Located primarily in back, leg, or both?
- Constant or intermittent?
- How do these symptoms limit you?
- How long can you sit, stand, walk?
- How much weight can you lift?
- When did the current limitations begin?

- How long have your activities been limited? More than 4 weeks?
- Have you had similar episodes previously?
- Previous testing or treatment?
- What do you hope we can accomplish during this visit?

❖ Physical Examination

Guided by the medical history, the physical examination includes:

- General observation of the patient.
- A regional back exam.
- Neurologic screening.
- Testing for sciatic nerve root tension.

The examination is mostly subjective since patient response or interpretation is required for all parts except reflex testing and circumferential measurements for atrophy.

Addressing Red Flags

Physical examination evidence of severe neurologic compromise that correlates with the medical history may indicate a need for immediate consultation. The examination may further modify suspicions of tumor, infection, or significant trauma. A medical history suggestive of non- spinal pathology mimicking a back problem may warrant examination of pulses, abdomen, pelvis, or other areas.

Observation and Regional Back Examination

Limping or coordination problems indicate the need for specific neurologic testing. Severe guarding of lumbar motion in all planes may support a suspected diagnosis of spinal infection, tumor, or fracture. However, given marked variations among persons with and without symptoms, range-of-motion measurements of the back are of limited value.

Vertebral point tenderness to palpation, when associated with other signs or symptoms, may be suggestive of but not specific for spinal fracture or infection. Palpable soft-tissue tenderness is, by itself, an even less specific or reliable finding.

Neurologic Screening

The neurologic examination can focus on a few tests that seek evidence of nerve root impairment, peripheral neuropathy, or spinal cord dysfunction. Over 90 percent of all clinically significant lower extremity radiculopathy due to disc herniation involves the L5 or S1 nerve root at the L4-5 or L5-S1 disc level. Features of nerve root compression are summarized below.

Figure 1. Testing for lumbar nerve root compromise.

Nerve root	L4	L5	S1
Pain	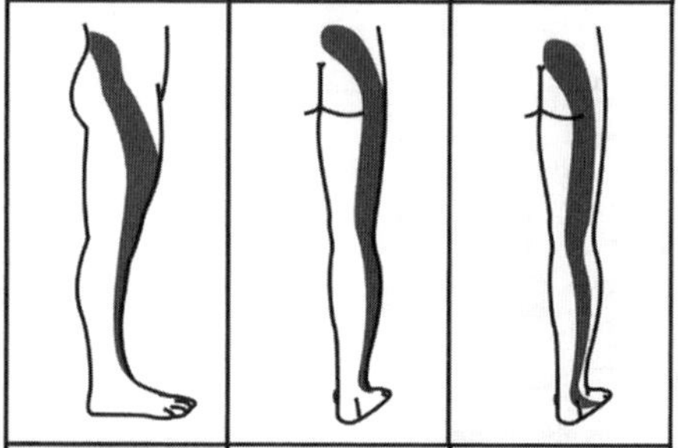		
Numbness	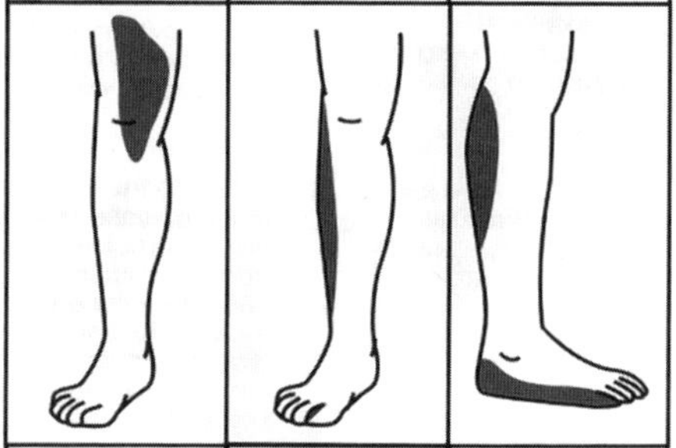		
Motor weakness	Extension of quadriceps.	Dorsilflexion of great toe and foot.	Plantar flexion of great toe and foot.
Screening exam	Squat & rise.	Heel walking.	Walking on toes.
Reflexes	Knee jerk diminished.	None reliable.	Ankle jerk diminished.

Testing for Muscle Strength

The patient's inability to toe walk (calf muscles, mostly S1 nerve root), heel walk (ankle and toe dorsiflexor muscles, L5 and some L4 nerve roots), or do a single squat and rise (quadriceps muscles, mostly L4 nerve root) may indicate muscle weakness. Specific testing of the dorsiflexor muscles of the ankle or great toe (suggestive of L5 or some L4 nerve root dysfunction), hamstrings and ankle evertors (L5-S1), and toe flexors (S1) is also important.

Circumferential Measurements

Muscle atrophy can be detected by circumferential measurements of the calf and thigh bilaterally. Differences of less than 2 cm in measurements of the two limbs at the same level may be a normal variation. Symmetrical muscle bulk and strength are expected unless the patient has a neurologic impairment or a history of lower extremity muscle or joint problem.

Reflexes

The ankle jerk reflex tests mostly the S1 nerve root and the knee jerk reflex tests mostly the L4 nerve root; neither tests the L5 nerve root. The reliability of reflex testing can be diminished in the presence of adjacent joint or muscle problems. Up-going toes in response to stroking the plantar footpad (Babinski or plantar response) may indicate upper motor-neuron abnormalities (such as myelopathy or demyelinating disease) rather than a common low back problem.

Sensory Examination

Testing light touch or pressure in the medial (L4), dorsal (L5), and lateral (S1) aspects of the foot (Figure 1)4 is usually sufficient for sensory screening.

Clinical Tests For Sciatic Tension

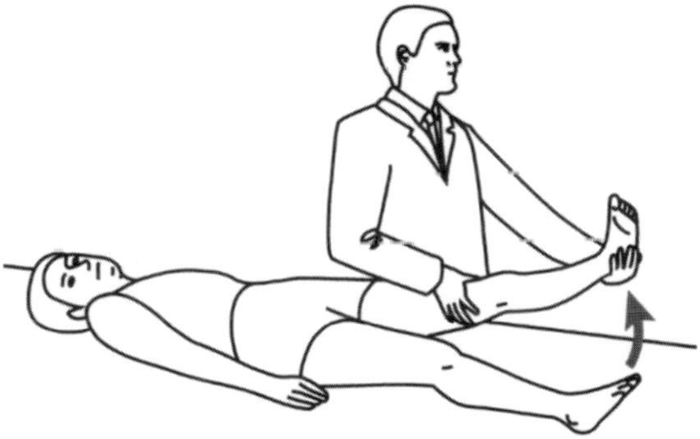

The straight leg raising (SLR) test can detect tension on the L5 and/or S1 nerve root. SLR may reproduce leg pain by stretching nerve roots irritated by a disc herniation. (1)Ask the patient to lie as straight as possible on a table in the supine position. (2) With one hand placed above the knee of the leg being examined, exert enough firm pressure to keep the knee fully extended. Ask the patient to relax.

(3) With the other hand cupped under the heel, slowly raise the straight limb. Tell the patient, "If this bothers you, let me know, and I will stop."

(4) Monitor for any movement of the pelvis before complaints are elicited. True sciatic tension should elicit complaints before the hamstrings are stretched enough to move the pelvis.

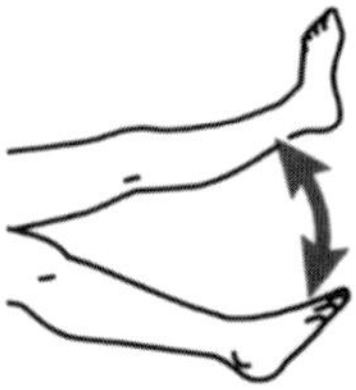

(5) Estimate the degree of leg elevation that elicits complaint from the patient. Then determine the most distal area of discomfort: back, hip, thigh, knee, or below the knee.

(6) While holding the leg at the limit of straight leg raising, dorsiflex the ankle. Note whether this aggravates the pain. Internal rotation of the limb can also increase the tension on the sciatic nerve roots.

Pain below the knee at less than 70 degrees of straight leg raising, aggravated by dorsiflexion of the ankle and relieved by ankle plantar flexion or external limb rotation, is most suggestive of tension on the L5 or S1 nerve root related to disc herniation. Reproducing back pain alone with SLR testing does not indicate significant nerve root tension.

Crossover pain occurs when straight raising of the patient's well limb elicits pain in the leg with sciatica. Crossover pain is a stronger indication of nerve root compression than pain elicited from raising the straight painful limb.

Sitting knee extension can also test sciatic tension. The patient with significant nerve root irritation tends to complain or lean backward to reduce tension on the nerve.

With the patient sitting on a table, both hip and knees flexed at 90 degrees, slowly extend the knee as if evaluating the patella or bottom of the foot. This maneuver stretches nerve roots as much as a moderate degree of supine SLR.

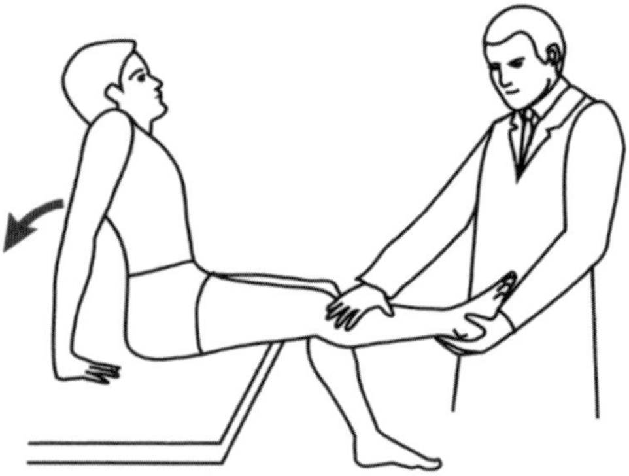

Algorithm 1.
Initial evaluation of acute low back problem

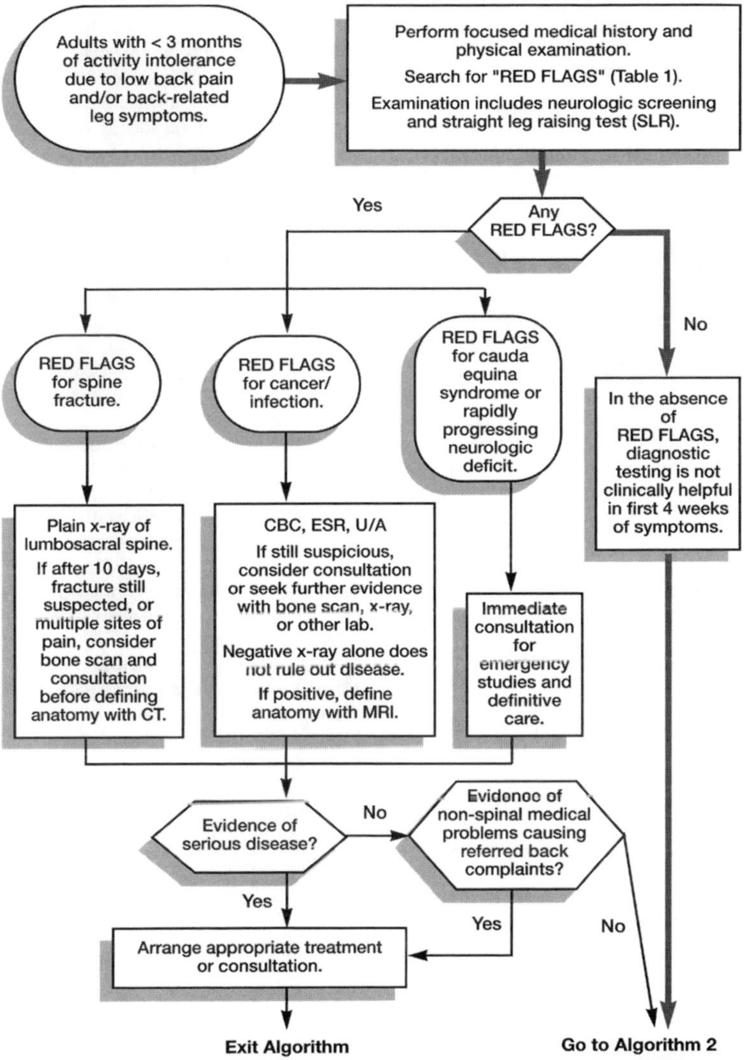

Inconsistent Findings and Pain Behavior

The patient who embellishes a medical history, exaggerates pain drawings, or provides responses on physical examination inconsistent with known physiology can be particularly challenging. A strongly positive supine straight leg raising test without complaint on sitting knee extension and inconsistent responses on examination raise a suspicion that nonphysical factors may be affecting the patient's responses. "Pain behaviors" (verbal or nonverbal communication of distress or suffering) such as amplified grimacing, distorted gait or posture, moaning, and rubbing of painful body parts may also cloud medical issues and even evoke angry responses from the clinician.

Interpreting inconsistencies or pain behaviors as malingering does not benefit the patient or the clinician. It is more useful to view such behavior and inconsistencies as the patient's attempt to enlist the practitioner as an advocate, a plea for help. The patient could be trapped in a job where activity requirements are unrealistic relative to the person's age or health. In some cases, the patient may be negotiating with an insurer or be involved in legal actions. In patients with recurrent back problems, inconsistencies and amplifications may simply be habits learned during previous medical evaluations. In working with these patients, the clinician should attempt to identify any psychological or socioeconomic pressures that might be influenced in a positive manner. The overall goal should always be to facilitate the patient's recovery and avoid the development of chronic low back disability.

❖ Initial Care

- Education and assurance. Patient comfort. Activity alterations.

Patient Education

If the initial assessment detects no serious condition, assure the patient that there is "no hint of a dangerous problem" and that "a rapid recovery can be expected." The need for education will vary among patients and during various stages of care. An obviously apprehensive patient may require a more detailed explanation. Patients with sciatica may have a longer expected recovery time than patients with nonspecific back symptoms and thus may need more education and reassurance. Any patient who does not recover within a few weeks may need more extensive education about back problems and the reassurance that special studies may be considered if recovery is slow.

Patient Comfort

Comfort is often a patient's first concern. Nonprescription analgesics will provide sufficient pain relief for most patients with acute low back symptoms. If treatment response is inadequate, as evidenced by continued symptoms and activity limitations, prescribed pharmaceuticals or physical methods may be added. Comorbid conditions, side effects, cost, and provider/patient preference should guide the clinician's choice of recommendations.

Oral Pharmaceuticals

The safest effective medication for acute low back problems appears to be acetaminophen. Nonsteroidal anti-inflammatory drugs (NSAIDs), including aspirin and ibuprofen, are also effective although they can cause gastrointestinal irritation/ulceration or (less commonly) renal or allergic problems. Phenylbutazone is not recommended due to risks of bone marrow suppression. Acetaminophen may be used safely in combination with NSAIDs or other pharmacological or physical therapeutics, especially in otherwise healthy patients.

Muscle relaxants seem no more effective than NSAIDs for treating patients with low back symptoms, and using them in combination with NSAIDs has no demonstrated benefit. Side effects including drowsiness have been reported in up to 30 percent of patients taking muscle relaxants.

Opioids appear no more effective than safer analgesics for managing low back symptoms. Opioids should be avoided if possible and, when chosen, used only for a short time. Poor patient tolerance and risks of drowsiness, decreased reaction time, clouded judgment, and potential misuse/dependence have been reported in up to 35 percent of patients. Patients should be warned of these potentially debilitating problems.

Table 2. Symptom Control Methods

1. Aspirin and other NSAIDs are not recommended for use in combination with one another due to the risk of GI complications.

2. Equivocal efficacy.

3. Significant potential for producing drowsiness and debilitation; potential for dependency.

4. Short course (few days only) for severe symptoms.

Physical Methods

Manipulation, defined as manual loading of the spine using short or long leverage methods, is safe and effective for patients in the first month of acute low back symptoms without radiculopathy. For patients with symptoms lasting longer than 1 month, manipulation is probably safe but its efficacy is unproven. If manipulation has not resulted in symptomatic and functional improvement after 4 weeks, it should be stopped and the patient reevaluated.

Traction applied to the spine has not been found effective for treating acute low back symptoms.

Physical modalities such as massage, diathermy, ultrasound, cutaneous laser treatment, biofeedback, and transcutaneous electrical nerve stimulation (TENS) also have no proven efficacy in the treatment of acute low back symptoms. If requested, the clinician may wish to provide the patient with instructions on self-application of heat or cold therapy for temporary symptom relief.

Invasive techniques such as needle acupuncture and injection procedures (injection of trigger points in the back; injection of facet joints; injection of steroids, lidocaine, or opioids in the epidural space) have no proven benefit in the treatment of acute low back symptoms.

Other miscellaneous therapies have been evaluated. No evidence indicates that shoe lifts are effective in treating acute low back symptoms or limitations, especially when the difference in lower limb length is less than 2 cm. Shoe insoles are a safe and inexpensive option if requested by patients with low back symptoms who must stand for prolonged periods. Low back corsets and back belts, however, do not appear beneficial for treating acute low back symptoms.

Activity Alteration

To avoid both undue back irritation and debilitation from inactivity, recommendations for alternate activity can be helpful. Most patients will not require bed rest. Prolonged bed rest (more than 4 days) has potential debilitating effects, and its efficacy in the treatment of acute low back problems is unproven. Two to four days of bed rest are reserved for patients with the most severe limitations (due primarily to leg pain).

- **Avoiding Undue Back Irritation**

Activities and postures that increase stress on the back also tend to aggravate back symptoms. Patients limited by back symptoms can minimize the stress of lifting by keeping any lifted object close to the body at the level of the navel. Twisting, bending, and reaching while lifting also increase stress on the back. Sitting, although safe, may aggravate symptoms for some patients. Advise these patients to avoid prolonged sitting and to change position often. A soft support placed at the small of the back, armrests to support some body weight, and a slight recline of the chair back may make required sitting more comfortable.

- **Avoiding Debilitation**

Until the patient returns to normal activity, aerobic (endurance) conditioning exercise such as walking, stationary biking, swimming, and even light jogging may be recommended to help avoid debilitation from inactivity. An incremental, gradually increasing regimen of aerobic exercise (up to 20 to 30 minutes daily) can usually be started within the first 2 weeks of symptoms. Such conditioning activities have been found to stress the back no more than sitting for an equal time period on the side of the bed. Patients should be informed that exercise may increase symptoms slightly at first. If intolerable, some exercise alteration is usually helpful.

Conditioning exercises for trunk muscles are more mechanically stressful to the back than aerobic exercise. Such exercises are not recommended during the first few weeks of symptoms, although they may later help patients regain and maintain activity tolerance.

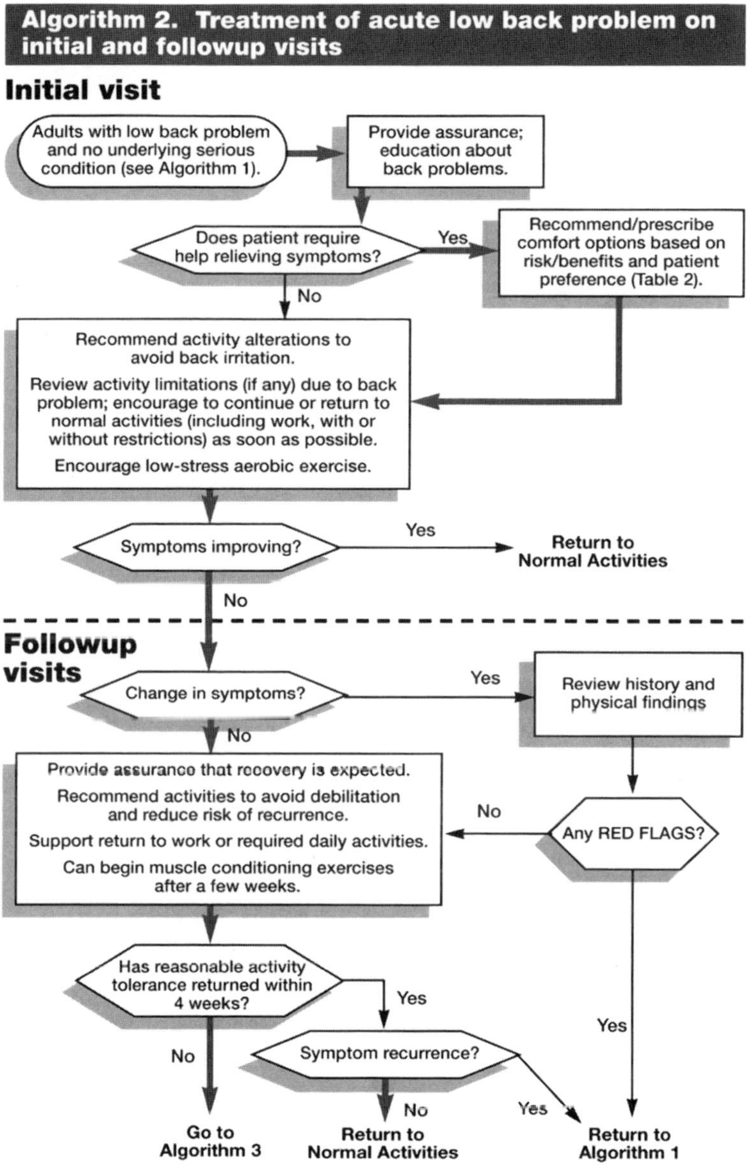

There is no evidence to indicate that back-specific exercise machines are effective for treating acute low back problems. Neither is there evidence that stretching of the back helps patients with acute symptoms.

Work Activities

When requested, clinicians may choose to offer specific instructions about activity at work for patients with acute limitations due to low back symptoms. The patient's age, general health, and perceptions of safe limits of sitting, standing, walking or lifting (noted on initial history) can help provide reasonable starting points for activity recommendations. Table 38 provides a guide for recommendations about sitting and lifting. The clinician should make clear to patients and employers that:

- Even moderately heavy unassisted lifting may aggravate back symptoms.
- Any restrictions are intended to allow for spontaneous recovery or time to build activity tolerance through exercise.

Activity restrictions are prescribed for a short time period only, depending upon work requirements (no benefits apparent beyond 3 months).

Table 3. Guidelines For Sitting And Unassisted Lifting

1 Without getting up and moving around.

2 Modification of NIOSH Lifting Guidelines, 1981, 1993. Gradually increase unassisted lifting limits to 60 lbs (men) and 35 lbs (women) by 3 months even with continued symptoms. Limit twisting, bending, and reaching. Always lift close to belly button.

Special Studies and Diagnostic Considerations

Routine testing (laboratory tests, plain x-rays of the lumbosacral spine) and imaging studies are not recommended during the first month of activity limitation due to back symptoms except when a red flag noted on history or examination raises suspicion of a dangerous low back or non- spinal condition. If a patient's limitations due to low back symptoms do not improve in 4 weeks, reassessment is recommended. After again reviewing the patient's activity limitations, history, and physical findings, the clinician may then consider further diagnostic studies, and discuss these with the patient.

❖ Timing and Limits of Special Studies

Waiting four weeks before considering special tests allows 90 percent of patients to recover spontaneously and avoids unneeded procedures. This also reduces the potential confusion of falsely labeling age-related changes on imaging studies (commonly noted in patients older than 30 without back symptoms) as the cause of the acute symptoms. In the absence of either red flags or persistent activity limitations due to continuous limb symptoms, imaging studies (especially plain x-rays) rarely provide information that changes the clinical approach to the acute low back problem.

Selection of Special Studies

Prior to ordering imaging studies the clinician should have noted either of the following:

- The emergence of a red flag.
- Physiologic evidence of tissue insult or neurological dysfunction.

Physiologic evidence may be in the form of definitive nerve findings on physical examination, electrodiagnostic studies (when evaluating sciatica), and a laboratory test or bone scan (when evaluating nonspecific low back symptoms). Unquestionable findings that identify specific nerve root compromise on the neurologic examination (see Figure 1) are sufficient physiologic evidence to warrant imaging. When the neurologic examination is less clear, however, further physiologic evidence of nerve root dysfunction should be considered before ordering an imaging study. Electromyography (EMG) including H-reflex tests may be useful to identify subtle focal neurologic dysfunction in patients with leg symptoms lasting longer than 3-4 weeks. Sensory evoked potentials (SEPs) may be added to the assessment if spinal stenosis or spinal cord myelopathy is suspected.

Laboratory tests such as erythrocyte sedimentation rate (ESR), complete blood count (CBC), and urinalysis (UA) can be useful to screen for nonspecific medical diseases (especially infection and tumor) of the low back. A bone scan can detect physiologic reactions to suspected spinal tumor, infection, or occult fracture.

Should physiologic evidence indicate tissue insult or nerve impairment, discuss with a consultant selection of an imaging test to define a potential anatomic cause (CT for bone, MRI for neural or other soft tissue). Anatomic definition is commonly needed to guide surgery or specific procedures. Selection of an imaging test should also take into consideration any patient allergies to contrast media (myelogram) or concerns about claustrophobia (MRI) and costs. A discussion with a specialist on selection of the most clinically valuable study can often assist the primary care clinician to avoid duplication.

In general, an imaging study may be an appropriate consideration for the patient whose limitations due to consistent symptoms have persisted for 1 month or more:

- When surgery is being considered for treatment of a specific detectable loss of neurological function.
- To further evaluate potentially serious spinal pathology.

Reliance upon imaging studies alone to evaluate the source of low back symptoms, however, carries a significant risk of diagnostic confusion, given the possibility of falsely identifying a finding that was present before symptoms began.

Algorithm 3. Evaluation of the slow-to-recover patient (symptoms > 4 weeks)

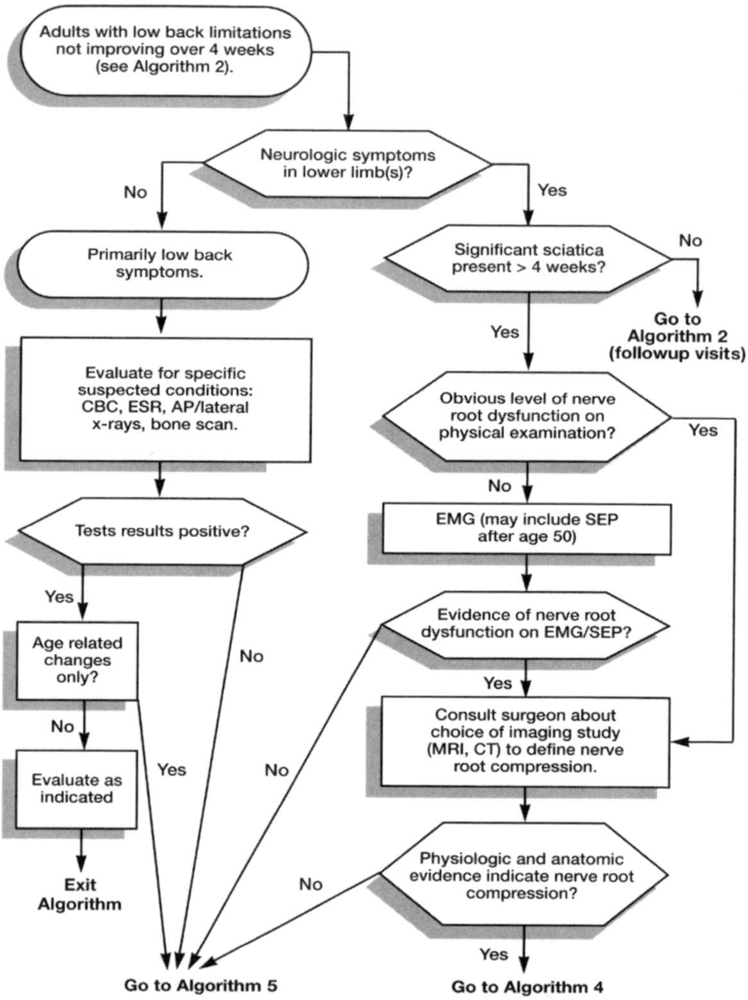

Table 4. Ability of Different Techniques To Identify And Define Pathology

1 Risk of complications (radiation, infection, etc.): highest for myelo- CT, second highest for myelography, and relatively less risk for bone scan, x-ray, and CT.

2 False-positive diagnostic findings in up to 30 percent of people without symptoms at age 30.

❖ Management Considerations After Special Studies

Definitive treatment for serious conditions detected by special studies is beyond the scope of this guideline. When special studies fail to define the exact cause of symptoms, however, no patient should receive an impression that the clinician thinks "nothing is wrong" or that the problem could be "in their head." Assure the patient that a clinical workup is highly successful in detecting serious conditions, but does not reveal the precise cause of most low back symptoms.

Surgical Considerations

Within the first 3 months of acute low back symptoms, surgery is considered only when serious spinal pathology or nerve root dysfunction obviously due to a herniated lumbar disc is detected. A disc herniation, characterized by protrusion of the central nucleus pulposus through a defect in the outer annulus fibrosis, may trap a nerve root causing irritation, leg symptoms and nerve root dysfunction. The presence of a herniated lumbar disc on an imaging study, however, does not necessarily imply nerve root dysfunction. Studies of asymptomatic adults commonly demonstrate intervertebral disc herniations that apparently do not entrap a nerve root or cause symptoms.

Therefore, nerve root decompression can be considered for a patient if all of the following criteria exist:

- Sciatica is both severe and disabling.
- Symptoms of sciatica persist without improvement for longer than 4 weeks or with extreme progression.
- There is strong physiologic evidence of dysfunction of a specific nerve root with inter-vertebral disc herniation confirmed at the corresponding level and side by findings on an imaging study.

Algorithm 4. Surgical considerations for patients with persistent sciatica

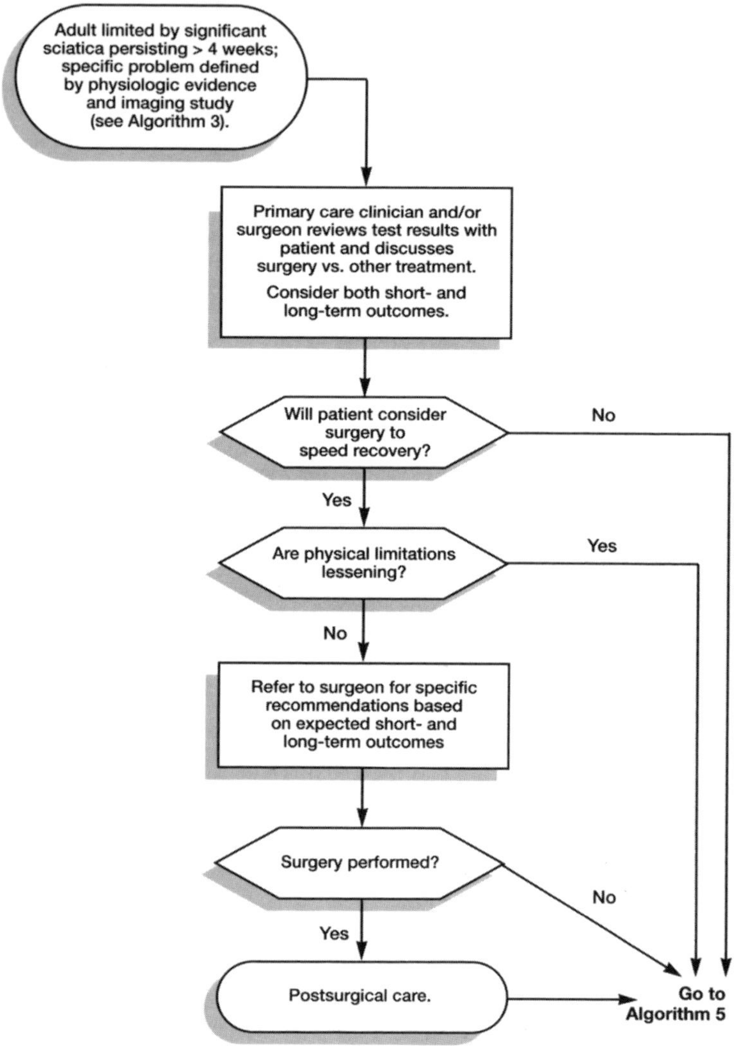

Patients with acute low back pain alone, without findings of serious conditions or significant nerve root compression, rarely benefit from a surgical consultation.

Many patients with strong clinical findings of nerve root dysfunction due to disc herniation recover activity tolerance within 1 month; no evidence indicates that delaying surgery for this period worsens outcomes. With or without an operation, more than 80 percent of patients with obvious surgical indications eventually recover. Surgery seems to be a luxury for speeding recovery of patients with obvious surgical indications but benefits fewer than 40 percent of patients with questionable physiologic findings. Moreover, surgery increases the chance of future procedures with higher complication rates. Overall, the incidence of first-time disc surgery complications, including infection and bleeding, is less than 1 percent. The figure increases dramatically with older patients or repeated procedures.

Direct And Indirect Nerve Root Decompression For Herniated Discs

Direct methods of nerve root decompression include laminotomy (expansion of the interlaminar space for access to the nerve root and the offending disc fragments), microdiscectomy (laminotomy using a microscope), and laminectomy (total removal of laminae). Methods of indirect nerve root decompression include chemonucleolysis, the injection of chymopapain or other enzymes to dissolve the inner disc. Such chemical treatment methods are less efficacious than standard or microdiscectomy and have rare but serious complications. Any of these methods is preferable to percutaneous discectomy (indirect, mechanical disc removal through a lateral disc puncture).

Management of Spinal Stenosis

Usually resulting from soft tissue and bony encroachment of the spinal canal and nerve roots, spinal stenosis typically has a gradual onset and begins in older adults. It is characterized by nonspecific limb symptoms, called ***neurogenic claudication*** or ***pseudoclaudication,*** that interfere with the duration of comfortable standing and walking. The symptoms are commonly bilateral and rarely associated with strong focal findings on examination. Neurogenic claudication, however, can be confused or coexist with ***vascular claudication,*** in which leg pain also limits walking. The symptoms of vascular insufficiency can be relieved by simply standing still while relief of neurogenic claudication symptoms usually require the patient to flex the lumbar spine or sit.

The surgical treatment for spinal stenosis is usually complete laminectomy for posterior decompression. Offending soft tissue and osteophytes that encroach upon nerve roots in the central spinal canal and foramen are removed. Fusion may be considered to stabilize a degenerative spondylolisthesis with motion between the slipped vertebra and adjacent vertebrae. Elderly patients with spinal stenosis who tolerate their daily activities usually need no surgery unless they develop new signs of bowel or bladder dysfunction. Decisions on treatment should take into account the patient's preference, lifestyle, other medical problems, and risks of surgery. Surgery for spinal stenosis is rarely considered in the first 3 months of symptoms.

Except for cases of trauma-related spinal fracture or dislocation, fusion alone is not usually considered in the first 3 months following onset of low back symptoms.

❖ Further Management Consideration

Following diagnostic or surgical procedures, the management of most patients becomes focused on improving physical conditioning through an incrementally increased exercise program. The goal of this program is to build activity tolerance and overcome individual limitations due to back symptoms. At this point in treatment, symptom control methods are only an adjunct to making prescribed exercises more tolerable.

- Begin with low-stress aerobic activities to improve general stamina (walking, riding a bicycle, swimming, and eventually jogging).
- Exercises to condition specific trunk muscles can be added a few weeks after. The back muscles may need to be in better condition than before the problem occurred. Otherwise, the back may continue to be painful and easily irritated by even mild activity. Following back surgery, recovery of activity tolerance may be delayed until protective muscles are conditioned well enough to compensate for any remaining structural changes.
- Finally, specific training to perform activities required at home or work can begin. The objective of this program is to increase the patient's tolerance in carrying out actual daily duties.
- When patients demonstrate difficulty regaining the ability to tolerate the activities they are required (or would like) to do, the clinician may pose the following diagnostic and treatment questions:
- Could the patient have a serious, undetected medical condition? A careful review of the medical history and physical examination is warranted.
- Are the patient's activity goals realistic? Exploring briefly the patient's expectations, both short- and long-term, of being able to perform specific activities at home, work, or recreation may help the patient assess whether such activity levels are actually achievable.
- If for any reason the achievement of activity goals seems unlikely, what are the patient's remaining options? To answer this question, the patient is often required to gather specific information from family, friends, employers, or others. If, on follow-up visits, the patient has made no effort to gather such information, the clinician has the opportunity to point out that low back symptoms alone rarely prevent a patient from addressing questions so important to his or her future. This observation can lead to an open, nonjudgmental discussion of common but complicated psychosocial problems or other issues that often can interfere with a patient's recovery from low back problems. The clinician can then help the patient address or

arrange further evaluation of any specific problem limiting the patient's progress. This can usually be accomplished as the patient continues, with the clinician's encouragement, to build activity tolerance through safe, simple exercises.

Algorithm 5. Further management of acute low back problem

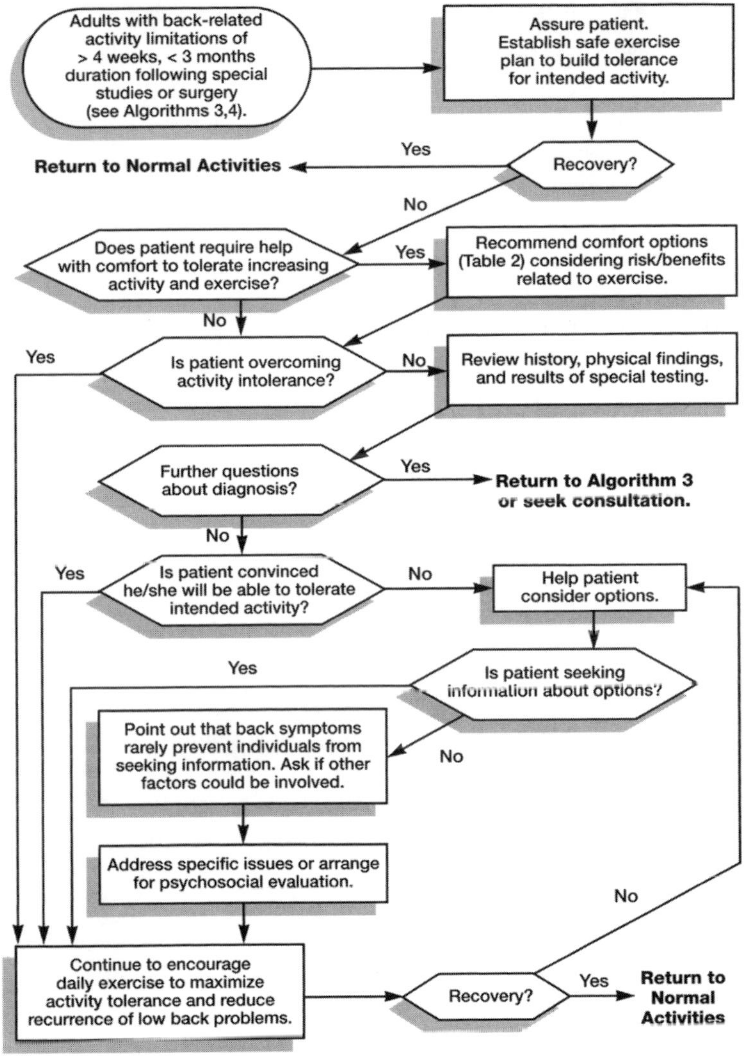

Table 5. Summary of Guideline Recommendations

The ratings in parentheses indicate the scientific evidence supporting each recommendation according to the following scale:

> A = strong research-based evidence (multiple relevant and high-quality scientific studies).
>
> B = moderate research-based evidence (one relevant, high-quality scientific study or multiple adequate scientific studies).
>
> C = limited research-based evidence (at least one adequate scientific study in patients with low back pain).
>
> D = panel interpretation of evidence not meeting inclusion criteria for research-based evidence.

The number of studies meeting panel review criteria is noted for each category.

Availability of Guidelines

For each clinical practice guideline developed under the sponsorship of the Agency for Health Care Policy and Research (AHCPR), several versions are produced to meet different needs.

The Clinical Practice Guideline presents recommendations for health care providers with brief supporting information, tables and figures, and pertinent references.

The Quick Reference Guide for Clinicians is a distilled version of the *Clinical Practice Guideline* summary points for ready reference on a day-to-day basis.

The Consumer Version, available in English and Spanish, is an information booklet for the general public to increase patient knowledge and involvement in health care decision making.

To order single copies of guideline products or to obtain further information on their availability, call the AHCPR Publications Clearinghouse toll-free at 800-358-9295 or write to: AHCPR Publications Clearinghouse, P.O. Box 8547, Silver Spring, MD 20907.

Single copies of the *Clinical Practice Guideline* are available for sale from the Government Printing Office, Superintendent of Documents, Washington, DC 20402, with a 25 percent discount given for bulk orders of 100 copies of more. The *Quick Reference Guide for Clinicians* and the *Consumer Version* in English are also available for sale in bulk quantities only. Call (202) 512-1800 for price and ordering information.

The *Guideline Technical Report* contains complete supporting materials for the *Clinical Practice Guideline*, including background information, methodology, literature review, scientific evidence tables, recommendations for research, and a comprehensive bibliography. It is available from the National Technical Information Service, 5285 Port Royal Road, Springfield, VA 22161. Call (703) 487-4650 for price and ordering information.

The full text of guideline documents for online retrieval may be accessed through a free, electronic service from the National Library of Medicine called HSTAT (Health Services/Technology Assessment Text). Guideline information is also available through some of the computer- based information systems of the National Technical Information Service, professional associations, nonprofit organizations, and commercial enterprises.

A fact sheet describing online access for *Clinical Practice Guidelines* (AHCPR Publication No. 94-0075) and copies of the *Quick Reference Guide for Clinicians* and the *Consumer Version* of each guideline are available through AHCPR's InstantFAX, a fax-on-demand service that operates 24 hours a day, 7 days a week. AHCPR's InstantFAX is accessible to anyone using a facsimile machine equipped with a touchtone telephone handset: Dial (301) 594-2800, push "1," and then press the facsimile machine's start button for instructions and a list of currently available publications.

U.S. Department of Health and Human Services, Public Health Service Agency for Health Care Policy and Research, Executive Office Center, Suite 501 2101 East Jefferson Street, Rockville, MD 20852 AHCPR Publication No. 95-0643 December 1994.

Appendix B

References and Recommended Reading

Internet Sites

www.chiromed.org
The National Association for Chiropractic Medicine Web site)

www.quackwatch.com
(A consumer-friendly, content-rich Web site that exposes health scams)

www.chirobase.org
A skeptical guide to chiropractic history, theories and current practices)

www.ncahf.org
(The National Council Against Health Fraud Web site, dedicated to promoting reliable health information)

www.healthwatcher.net
(A Canadian Web site dedicated to exposing health scams)

www.bmj.com
(A clearinghouse for medical information)

www.mailbase.ac.uk/lists
- then click on Health and then on Evidence Based Health (A British Web site that includes at least 31 articles on evidence-based health care)

www.ahcpr.gov
(The Web site for the Agency for Healthcare Research and Quality)

www.nccam.nih.gov
The Web site for the National Institutes of Health National Center for Complementary and Alternative Medicine--read this with a skeptical mindset)

Books

Roland, Professor Martin. (1996) The Back Book. United Kingdom: The Stationery Office Books. Available through www.amazon.co.uk

Bigos, S., Bowyer, O, Braen, G., et al. (December 1994) Acute Low Back Problems in Adults. Washington: U.S. Department of Health and Human Services, Agency for Healthcare Research and Quality, Pub. No. 95-0643.

Chapman-Smith, David. (2000) The Chiropractic Profession. West Des Moines, Ia: NCMIC Group, Inc.

Sarno, John M.D. (1999) Mind Over Back Pain. New York: Berkley Publishing Group.

Chotkowski, L.A., M.D. (1998) Chiropractic: The Greatest Hoax of the Century? Kensington, Conn.: New England Novelty Books.

Homola, Samuel D.C. (1999). Inside Chiropractic: A Patient's Guide. Buffalo: Prometheus Books.

Schaefer, R.C., D.C. and Sportelli, Louis D.C. (1994). Opportunities in Chiropractic Health- Care Careers. Lincolnwood, Ill.: Vgm Career Horizons.

Humber, James M. and Almeder, Robert F. (1998). Alternative Medicine and Ethics. Totowa, N.J.: Humana Press.

Magner, George. (1995). Chiropractic: The Victim's Perspective. Buffalo: Prometheus Books.

Sarno, John M.D. (1991). Healing Back Pain: The Mind-Body Connection. New York: Warner Books.

Dawes, Martin.(1999), Evidence-Based Practice: A Primer for Health Care Professionals. New York: Churchill Livingstone.

Maurer, Edward L. Selected Ethics and Protocols in Chiropractic. Gaithersburg, Md: Aspen Publishers, Inc.,.

Spencer, John Ph.D. (1983). Complementary/Alternative Medicine: An Evidence-Based Approach. St. Louis: Mosby – Year Book.

Starr, Paul. (1982). The Social Transformation of American Medicine. Basic Books.

Fuchs, Victor. (1998). Who Shall Live? River Edge, N.J.: World Scientific Publishing Company.

Articles

Brunette, D.M. Ph.D. (1997). "Alternative Therapies: Abuses of Scientific Method and Challenges to Dental Research." Journal of Prosthetic Dentistry, Vo. 80, No. 5, pp. 605-613.

Rosner, Anthony L., Ph.D. (1996). "The Role of Subluxation in Chiropractic." Des Moines, Iowa: Foundation for Chiropractic Education and Research, 1997.

"Practice Guidelines for Straight Chiropractic." (1992). Chandler, Ariz.: World Chiropractic Alliance.

Barrett, Stephen M.D. (2000). "Chiropractic's Elusive Subluxation." www.quackwatch.com

Peterson, Donald M. Jr. (2000). "NCC Raises the Admission Standard." Dynamic Chiropractic, Vol. 17, No. 20, pp. 1 and 38.

"Position Paper on Chiropractic." (Feb. 14, 1985). Loma Linda, Calif.: The National Council Against Health Fraud.

Pierse, Patrick M.D. (December 15, 1998). "Pediatricians Address Alberta Standing Committee on Health About Chiropractic Spending and Tactics." Edmonton, Alberta: Pediatric Alberta Medical Association, Vo. 2, No. 1, pp.5-6.

Nelson, Craig F., D.C. (1998). "Understanding Alternative Care." Journal of the Neuromusculoskeletal System, Vo. 6, No. 3.

Samanta, Ash.(April 24, 1999). "Low Back Pain: Which is the Best Way Forward?" British Medical Journal, pp. 1122-1123.

"Back Care."(1997). Rochester, Minn.: Mayo Clinic Health Letter, ISSN 0741-6245, pp. 1-8.

Schlosberg, Suzanne. (1999 July). "Exactly What Can Chiropractic Do For You Anyhow?" Shape Magazine, pp. 119-125.

French et al. (May, 2000). "Reliability of Chiropractic Methods Commonly Used to Detect Manipulable Lesions in Patients With Chronic Low Back Pain." Journal of Manipulative and Physiological Therapeutics, pp. 231-238.

Gottlieb, Scott. (October 17, 1998). "Chiropractic Treatment is of Limited Benefit." British Medical Journal, p. 1036.

Hansel and Slazak. (March 4, 1997) "Chiropractic Role in the Treatment of Disease." Journal of Manipulative and Physiological Therapeutics, Vol. 20, No. 3, pp. 220-223. "Chiropractic Rx Does Not Ease Tension Headache." (1998). Journal of the American Medical Association, Vo. 280: pp. 1576-1579.

Triano, John D.C. and Hansen, Daniel T. D.C. "Chiropractic and Quality Care: Are They Exclusive?" Journal of the Neuromusculoskeletal System, Vol. 7, No. 1, pp.25-33.

"Spinal Coupling Mechanics Part 2: Implications for Chiropractic Theories and Practice." Journal of Manipulative and Physiological Therapeutics, Vol. 21, No. 3, pp. 1-10.

Nelson, Craig F. D.C. "Spinal Manipulation and Chiropractic: Views of a Reformist Chiropractor. American Council on Science and Health, Vol. 11, No. 2, pp. 1-6.

"Scientific Monograph of the Quebec Task Force on Whiplash-Associated Disorders: Redefining Whiplash and its Management." Spine, Vol. 20, No. 8 S, pp. 25-68 S.

Khan, S. and Cook, J. (1999). "A Symptomatic Classification of Whiplash Injury and the Implications for Treatment." Journal of Orthopedic Medicine, Vo. 21, No. 1, pp. 21-25.

Pearce, Jules. (2000). "Aspects of the Failed Back Syndrome: Role of Litigation." Spinal Cord, Vol. 38, pp. 63-70..

Cassidy, David J. and Carroll, Linda J. "Effect of Eliminating Compensation for Pain and Suffering on the Outcome of Insurance Claims for Whiplash Injury." New England Journal of Medicine, Vol. 342, No. 16, pp. 1179-1186.

Fitz James, Michael. (July 4, 2000). "Law Journal Plays Hardball Over Whiplash Stats." Doctors and the Law, Vol. 36, No. 25.

Appendix C

Glossary

As typically seen in chiropractic, some of the terms in this glossary have as many diverse meanings as there are types of chiropractors and treatment techniques. The following definitions are consistent with my understanding of them and how they were used in this book. These are **consumer-friendly** definitions. These are working and operative definitions. They are not dictionary definitions as most of the time I have found those to be inadequate.

Acupuncture
... Used as an adjunct by many chiropractors, it consists of puncturing the skin at certain points, to promote healing. Acupressure is identical in scope, but the skin is not punctured, hoped for outcomes are similar.

Active care
... This type of care is performed by the patient. Examples would be aerobics, endurance exercises (weight lifting) and taking part in the health care decision-making process. It is what you do for yourself, not what someone does to you.

Acute back pain
... Short-term episodic pain in the back. From onset to 72 hours is the first stage, 72 hours to 6 weeks is the final stage. Most all back pain, regardless if treatment is rendered or not, will disappear during these phases.

Ad hominem
... An attack on a person and not on the message they delivered, express, or have. A childish and uneducated way to attack someone's ideas and thoughts.

AHCPR
... Agency for Health Care Policy and Research, part of the U. S. Department of Health and Human Services. Agency responsible for the Acute Low Back Pain in Adults Guideline and many others.

Alternative medicine
... Medicine not widely taught in western medical schools or practiced

in hospitals. I will suggest to you that the term should be dropped. Medicine is neither alternative or complementary in my opinion, either it is medicine that works or medicine that does not.

ACA
... American Chiropractic Association is the largest national association for chiropractors to belong to, comprised primarily of mixers.

Anecdotes
... Success stories used by chiropractors and their patients to recruit others. Entertaining, but at the bottom of the scientific pool of evidence. Never made a decision on health care because of an anecdote.

Arbitration
... A legal proceeding where attorneys present their cases to other attorneys instead of a judge and jury.

Aromatherapy
... The belief that certain smells and oils can cure disease or bring about relation.

Aura adjustment
... This attempts to treat the body's "aura" that surrounds it. It will be "treated" usually without any physical contact by the health care provider.

Board complaint
... A complaint filed usually by a patient against a chiropractor alleging wrongdoing. Used against me as a weapon to harass and discredit, never filed by a patient.

Capper
... A person who solicits accident victims for chiropractors and/or attorneys. Also can be called a runner.

CAM
... Complementary Alternative Medicine. Term should be dropped. Again, medicine either works or it does not.

CDE 1
... Certified Disability Examiner 1. One of three certifications through

the National Association of Disability Evaluating Professionals. Trained in a variety of examination techniques.

Charlatan
... A quack who makes money at it.

CFE
... Certified Fraud Examiner. An individual with the training to detect a variety of fraudulent schemes.

Chiropractic adjustment
... The main tool used to treat everything under the skin, by chiropractors of course.

Chronic
... Acute unresolved back pain beyond six weeks. Many, if not most, sources say beyond three months.

Clinical trials
... A type of research that investigates care and its outcome, not a story from a provider.

CGP
... Clinical Practice Guideline. A research set of information presented as a guideline to assist providers in making informed choices on patient care.

Consultant
... Acts as an advisor to interested parties.

Court reporter
... The person who types all the information and takes it down during legal proceedings.

Cult
... A group of charlatans.

Cytotechnology
... The study of cells, many times using an electron microscope.

Electrical Muscle Stimulation
... EMS is an electrical therapy that feels good and tingles, but does little, if anything, besides increase the provider's fees.

Evidence-based medicine
... EMB is the medicine based on the best available knowledge, not intuition, opinion or financial reward. The opposite of an anecdote.

Evidence-based practitioner
... A provider who knows of and practices evidence-based medicine.

Expert witness
... An individual who tries to educate juries, attorneys, and anyone else who is interested to the facts of the case at hand. A person who knows more and more about less and less, until finally they know everything about nothing.

Deposition
... Being asked questions under oath.

Diagnostic triage
... Determining which category a back pain patient falls into, mechanical, root, or serious. Most frequently heard of term in MASH episodes.

Fraud
... A willful attempt to deceive.

Full body x-rays
... Also known as full-spine x-rays. X-ray exposure of your body from head to pelvis, usually without lead shields protecting your eyes, thyroid or gonads.

HEAL
... Health Education Assistance Loan. Governmental loans that the chiropractic profession defaults on more than any other profession.

Herniated disk
... The disk separates your vertebra (back bones) from each other and they act as shock absorbers. A herniated disk can cause pain, but they are also routinely seen in backs without pain.

Herbalist
... Lay person or health care provider who use herbs as their panacea to cure you.

Homeopath
... Uses highly diluted solutions to treat your symptoms. No evidence to support this concept.

Hypermobility
... Back joints that move too much. They should not get manipulated or adjusted.

ICA
... International Chiropractic Association. A smaller version of the ACA. These groups of chiropractors are sincere believers in the subluxation.

Ice
... Use it as described and never be caught without your Styrofoam cup in the freezer.

IME
... Independent Medical Examination. An examination of a patient being treated by someone else and a report is generally authored containing the details of that examination.

Insurance adjustor
... An individual who reviews claims submitted by health care providers before payment is rendered.

Heat
... Use warm moist compresses to alleviate some types of back pain at home.

JMPT
... A peer-reviewed journal primarily written for and by chiropractors. Stands for Journal of Manipulative and Physiological Therapeutics.

Low-volt current
... Another type of electrical stimulation with the same hopes, desires and failures.

Malpositioned articulations
... Another fancy-sounding phrase for subluxations. The elusive subluxation dos not exist. Do not ever pay to have one corrected.

Mixers
... One of the many types of chiropractors, opposite of straights. This

group believes in electrical stimulation and other passive therapies and use them as complements to their adjustments.

Meta-analysis
... A way to look at a group of research studies and form an opinion.

Musculoskeletal
... The back, arms, legs, muscles, ligaments and tendons of your body.

Massage
... A formal back rub that feels good only. No curative value.

NACM
... National Association of Chiropractic Medicine. A scientific group of chiropractors who do not recognize or treat the elusive subluxation.

Natural history
... The course of a bad back whether treatment is rendered or not. Ninety-five percent of mechanical back pain, which makes up 98% of all bad backs, will get better without care in six weeks. If you seek care, do not go beyond four weeks with a chiropractor or any type of manipulation.

Naturopath
... Another CAM belief system. Forget about it.

NICB
... National Insurance Crime Bureau. They have a representative in your area. Call them if you suspect health fraud.

Neurologist
... Medical doctor who specializes in diseases of the nervous system.

National Center for Complementary and Alternative Medicine (NCCAM)
... An organization within the National Institute of Health researching CAM therapies and their therapeutic value.

NOOPE
... No out of pocket expense. If it sounds good, it probably isn't. Remember that old saying.

NSAID
... Non-steroidal anti-inflammatory drugs. Over-the-counter anti-inflammatory drugs commonly recommended for back pain relief.

Orthopedic technician
... An individual who assists orthopedic surgeons in and out of the operating room.

Orthopedists
... The original "saw bones." Practices "sterilized carpentry" on the musculoskeletal system.

Oncology
... The study and treatment of cancer.

P.A.I.N.E.D
... An acronym to assist you in relieving your back pain.

Panacea
... A belief that their approach to treatment is a cure-all for everything. Chiropractic can be used to treat everything through ridding your body of subluxations. There are no such things as panaceas.

Passive treatments
... The feel-good care that a patient passively receives. Cures nothing. Active care cures, do it yourself.

Peer review
... A document review of another doctor's patient chart or care requested by a third party.

Physical therapist
... A knowledgeable health care provider who does not routinely manipulate. Treats the entire human frame to rehabilitate and restore function.

Physical modalities
... Another name for the costly non-cure of passive therapies.

Plaintiff lawyer
... The attorney who seeks money from car accidents.

Placebo
... If you believe in your treatment, regardless of what it is, you will

probably get better. One study shows 35% of a treatments benefit is the therapeutic effect of placebo.

Primary care physician
... The family medical doctor.

Pseudo-science
... False science, spinned science, half-truth science. Used frequently in alternative medicine.

Quack
... An individual who aspires to be a charlatan. After reading this book, it is less probably that it will happen to you. Congratulations!

Radiculopathy
... Pain, numbness and tingling going into your buttock or down the back of your leg, even into your toes. The scientific term for "sciatica".

Sprain
... A separation of soft tissue, mainly ligaments. Moderate and severe sprains should not be manipulated in most cases. A severe sprain routinely requires surgery.

Strain
... Muscles only under an unusual load. Self-resolving many times and no care is required.

Straights
... Big-time subluxation believers. Opposite in many ways from the mixer group.

Stroke
... Can be a complication after a neck adjustment/manipulation. Can paralyze or kill the patient. One out of fifteen hundred to one out of millions is the occurrence rate, depending on the study. Be careful!

Spinal manipulation
... The chiropractor uses his hands to "crack" your back and hopefully not your ribs.

Subluxations
... From 1895 until now, there is no scientific proof that they exist, affect your health or can be defined universally within the profession. Another one of those "forget about it".

State Boards

... A panel of chiropractors and laypersons responsible for protecting consumers in that state.

Subpoena

... A legal document from the court requesting information. A court order.

Techniques

... A generic name for all of the hundreds of ways chiropractors will attempt to treat you and take your money.

Testimonials

... Stories/anecdotes about how well an individual chiropractor's technique works.

The Back Book

... The only evidence-based patient education booklet I know of. Excellence source of active knowledge. Get one.

Traction

... Can be manual or by lying on a table. Again, passive in nature so it feels good, but cures what?

Ultrasound

... Another passive therapy done properly you will not feel a thing. Messy, cold ... who cares?

Whiplash

... Neck pain allegedly caused by a car accident. The main source of chiropractic income.

Appendix D

State Boards of Chiropractic Examiners

ALABAMA STATE BOARD OF CHIROPRACTIC EXAMINERS

737 Logan Road; Clanton, AL 35045; Phone: 205-755-8000; Fax: 205-755-0081

ALASKA STATE BOARD OF CHRIOPRACTIC EXAMINERS

Division of Occupational Licensing; 333 Willoughby Avenue, 9th Floor; P.O. Box 110806; Juneau, AK 99811-0806; Phone: 907-465-2589; Fax: 907-465-2974;
E-mail: license@commerce.state.ak.us
Web: www.commerce.state.ak.us/occ/pchi

STATE OF ARIZONA BOARD OF CHIROPRACTIC EXAMINERS

5060 North 19th Avenue, Suite 416; Phoenix, AZ 850015;
Phone: 602-255-1444; Fax: 602-255-4289; E-mail: board@goodnet.com

ARKANSAS STATE BOARD OF CHIROPRACTIC EXAMINERS

101 East Capitol Street, Suite 209; Little Rock, AR 72201;
Phone: 501-682-9015; Fax: 501-682-9016

CALIFORNIA BOARD OF CHIROPRACTIC EXAMINERS

2710-N Gateway Oaks Drive, Suite 100; Sacramento, CA 95833-3505; Phone: 916-263-5355; Fax: 916-263-5369 Web: www.dca.ca.gov/r_chiropra.htm

COLORADA STATE BOARD OF CHIROPRACTIC EXAMINERS

1560 Broadway, Suite 1310; Denver, CO 80202; Phone: 303-894-7758, Ext. 301;
Fax: 303-894-7764 Web: www.dora.state.co.us/chiropractic

CONNECTICUT STATE BOARD OF CHIROPRACTIC EXAMINERS

410 Capitol Avenue, MS#12APP; P.O. Box 340308; Hartford, CT 06134;
Phone: 860-509-7561; Fax: 860-509-8457 Web: www.state.ct.us/dph

DELAWARE BOARD OF CHIROPRACTIC

Division of Professional Regulation; Suite 203, Cannon Building; 861 Silver Lake Blvd.; Dover, DE 19904; Phone: 302-739-4522, Ext. 204;
Fax: 302-739-2711

GOVERNMENT OF THE DISTRICT OF COLUMBIA BOARD OF CHIROPRACTIC

614 H Street, N.W., Room 108; Washington, D.C. 20001;
Phone: 202-727-5365; Fax: 202-727-4087

FLORIDA BOARD OF CHIROPRACTIC MEDICINE

Department of Health; 2020 Capital Circle SE, Bin #C07; Tallahassee, FL 32399-0752; Phone: 850-488-0595; Fax: 850-922-8876;
Web: www.doh.state.fl.us

GEORGIA BOARD OF CHIROPRACTIC EXAMINERS

166 Pryor Street, SW; Atlanta, GA 30303; Phone: 404-656-3912; Fax: 404-6574220; Web: www.sos.state.ga.us/ebd-chiro E-mail: clbarnes@sos.state.ga.us

HAWAII STATE BOARD OF CHIROPRACTIC EXAMINERS

Department of Commerce and Consumer Affairs; 1010 Richards Street; Honolulu, HI 96813; P.O. Box 3469; Honolulu, HI 96801;
Phone: 808-586-3000; E-mail: kyokouchi@ncsbn.org

IDAHO STATE BOARD OF CHIROPRACTIC PHYSICIANS

Bureau of Occupational Licenses; 1109 Main Street, Suite 220; Boise, ID 83702-5642; Phone: 208-334-3233; Fax: 208-334-3945;
E-mail: rswanbro@ibol.state.id.us

ILLINOIS MEDICAL LICENSING BOARD

Medical Licensing Unit; Department of Professional Regulation; 320 W. Washington, Third Floor; Springfield, IL 62786; Phone: 217-524-7534;
Fax: 217-524-2169; Web: www.state.il.us/dpr

INDIANA BOARD OF CHIROPRACTIC EXAMINERS

Health Professions Bureau; 402 West Washington Street; Room 041; Indianapolis, IN 46204; Phone: 317-233-4407; Fax: 317-233-4236;
E-mail: cvaught@hpb.state.in.us Web: www.ai.org/hbp/ibce

IOWA BOARD OF CHIROPRACTIC EXAMINERS

Department of Public Health; Lucas State Office Bldg, 4th Floor; 321 E 12th St; Des Moines, IA 50319-0075; Phone: 515-281-4416; Fax: 515-281-3121;
E-mail: sdozier@idph.state.ia.us

KANSAS STATE BOARD OF HEALING ARTS

235 South Topeka Boulevard; Topeka, KS 66603; Phone: 785-296-7413;
Fax: 785-296-0852; E-mail: cabbott@ink.org Web: www.ink.org/public/boha

KENTUCKY STATE BOARD OF CHIROPRACTIC EXAMINERS

P.O. Box 183; Glasgow, KY 42124-0183; Phone: 502-651-2522;
Fax: 502-651-8784; E-mail: kychiro@Glasgow-ky.com

LOUISIANA STATE BOARD OF CHIROPRACTIC EXAMINERS

8621 Summa Avenue; Baton Rouge, LA 70809; Phone: 225-765-2322;
Fax: 225-765-2640; E-mail: isbce@eatel.net

MAINE BOARD OF CHIROPRACTIC EXAMINATION & REGISTRATION

Department of Professional and Financial Regulation; State House Station 35;
Augusta, ME 04333; Phone: 207-624-8600;
Web: www.state.me.us/pfr/led/chiro.index.htm

MARYLAND BOARD OF CHIROPRACTIC EXAMINERS

Department of Health and Mental Hygiene; 4201 Patterson Avenue; Baltimore, Maryland 21215-2299; Phone: 410-764-4726; Fax: 410-358-1879

MASSACHUSETTS BOARD OF REGISTRATION OF CHIROPRACTORS

Leverett Saltonstall Building, Room 1513; 100 Cambridge Street; Boston, MA 02202; Phone: 617-727-3093; E-mail: internetmail@gateways;
Web: www.magnet.state.ma.us/reg/boards/ch/default.htm

MICHIGAN BOARD OF CHIROPRACTIC

611 West Ottawa; Lansing, MI 48933; Phone: 517-335-0918; Fax: 517-373-2179;
Web: www.cis.state.mi.us/ohs

MINNESOTA BOARD OF CHIROPRACTIC EXAMINERS

2829 University Avenue, SE-#300; Minneapolis, MN 55414-3220;
Phone: 612-617-2222; Fax: 612-617-2224; E-mail: larry.spicer@state.mn.us
Web: www.mn-chiroboard.state.mn.us

MISSISSIPPI STATE BOARD OF CHIROPRACTIC EXAMINERS

P.O. Box 775; Louisville, MS 39339; Phone: 601-773-4433; Fax: 601-773-4433

MISSOURI STATE BOARD OF CHIROPRACTIC EXAMINERS

3605 Missouri Boulevard; Jefferson City, MO 65109; Phone: 573-751-2104;
Fax: 573-751-0735; E-mail: chiro@mail.state.mo.us
Web: www.ecodev.state.mo.us/pr/chiro

MONTANA BOARD OF CHIROPRACTORS

Arcade Building; 111 North Jackson; P.O. Box 200513; Helena, MT 59620-0513; Phone: 406-444-5433; Fax: 406-444-1677; E-mail: cheryls@state.mt.us
Web: www.state.mt.us

NEBRASKA BOARD OF EXAMINERS IN CHIROPRACTIC

Nebraska Health and Human Services; Department of Regulation and Licensure; Rehabilitation & Community Services Section; 301 Centennial Mall South; P.O. Box 94986; Lincoln, NE 68509-4986; Phone: 402-471-2299; Fax: 402-471-3577; E-mail: doh6151@vmhost.cdp.state.ne.us Web: www.hhs.state.ne.us

CHIROPRACTIC PHYSICIANS' BOARD OF NEVADA

4600 Kietzke Lane; Suite M-245; Reno, NV 89502; Phone: 775-688-1919; Fax: 775-688-1920; E-mail: chirobd@govmail.state.nv.us
Web: www.state.nv.us/chirobd

NEW HAMPSHIRE BOARD OF CHIROPRACTIC EXAMINERS

Health & Welfare Building; 6 Hazen Drive; Concord, NH 03301-6527; Phone: 603-271-4560; Fax: 605-271-4827

NEW JERSEY STATE BOARD OF CHIROPRACTIC EXAMINERS

124 Halsey Street; P.O. Box 45004; Newark, NJ 07101; Phone: 973-504-6395; Fax: 973-648-2855; E-mail: earlek@smpt.lps.state.nj.us

NEW MEXICO BOARD OF CHIROPRACTIC EXAMINERS

2055 South Pacheco, Suite 400; P.O. Box 25101; Santa Fe, NM 87504; Phone: 505-476-7120; E-mail: RLDCB@state.nm.us

NEW YORK STATE BOARD FOR CHIROPRACTIC

Customer Service Unit, Division of Professional Licensing Services; Cultural Education Center, Room 3041; Albany, NY 12230; Phone: 518-486-3817; Fax: 518-486-2981; E-mail: chirobd@mail.nysed.gov
Web: www.nysed.gov/prof/profhome.htm

NORTH CAROLINA BOARD OF CHIROPRACTIC EXAMINERS

174 North Church Street; Concord, NC 28025; Phone: 704-793-1342; Fax: 704-793-1385; E-mail: ncchirobrd@juno.com Web: www.ncchiroboard.org

NORTH DAKOTA STATE BOARD OF CHIROPRACTIC EXAMINERS

Highway 17 West; P.O. Box 185; Grafton, ND 58237; Phone: 701-352-1690; Fax: 701-352-2258; E-mail: docJDC@polarcomm.com

OHIO STATE BOARD OF CHIROPRACTIC EXAMINERS

77 South High Street, 16th Floor; Columbus, OH 43266-0542; Phone: 614-644-7032; Fax: 614-752-2539; E-mail: chirobd@mail.peps.state.oh.us
Web: www.ohio.gov/chr

OKLAHOMA BOARD OF CHIROPRACTIC EXAMINERS

310 NE 28th, #205; Oklahoma City, OK 73105; Phone: 405-528-5505; Fax: 405-528-5447; E-mail: OBCEok@aol.com Web: www.oklaosf.state.ok.us

OREGON BOARD OF CHIROPRACTIC EXAMINERS

3218 Pringle Road SE, Suite 150; Salem, OR 97302-6311; Phone: 503-378-5816; Fax: 503-362-1260; E-mail: obce@state.or.us Web: www.obce.state.or.us

PENNSYLVANIA STATE BOARD OF CHIROPRACTIC

Department of State; 116 Pine Street, 5th Floor; P.O. Box 2649; Harrisburg, PA 17105-2649; Phone: 717-783-7155; Fax: 717-787-7769; E-mail: chiropa@pados.dos.state.pa.us Web: www.dos.state.pa.us/bpoa/chibd.htm

RHODE ISLAND BOARD OF EXAMINERS IN CHIROPRACTIC

Division of Professional Regulation; Three Capitol Hill, Room 104; Providence, RI 02908-5097; Phone: 401-222-2827; Fax: 401-222-1272

SOUTH CAROLINA BOARD OF CHIROPRACTIC EXAMINERS

110 Centerview Drive, Suite 306; Columbia, SC 29210; P.O. Box 11329; Columbia, SC 29211-1329; Phone: 803-896-4587; Fax: 803-896-4719; E-mail: holmesa@mail.llr.sc.us Web: www.LLR.STATE.SC.US

SOUTH DAKOTA BOARD OF CHIROPRACTIC EXAMINERS

1406 Mount Rushmore Road; Rapid City, SD 57701-4582; Phone: 605-343-7440; Fax: 605-342-7868; E-mail: sdbce@rapidnet.com
Web: www.state.sd.us/dcr/chiropractic

TENNESSEE BOARD OF CHIROPRACTIC EXAMINERS

425 5th Avenue, North, 1st Floor; Cordell Hull Building; Nashville, TN 37247-1010; Phone: 615-532-5096; Fax: 615-532-5369;
Web: www.state.tn.us/health/professions

TEXAS BOARD OF CHIROPRACTIC EXAMINERS

333 Guadeloupe, Tower III, Suite 815; Austin, TX 78701; Phone: 512-305-6700; Fax: 512-305-6705; E-mail: tbce@tbce.state.tx.us Web: www.tbce.state.tx.us

UTAH CHIROPRACTIC PHYSICIANS LICENSING BOARD

160 East 300 South; Box 146741; Salt Lake City, UT 84114-6741; Phone: 801-530-6623; Fax: 801-530-6511
Web: www.commerce.state.ut.us/web/commerce/DOPL/dopl1.htm

VERMONT BOARD OF CHIROPRACTIC

26 Terrace Street, Drawer 09; Montpelier, VT 05609-1101; Phone: 802-828-2390; Fax: 802-828-2465; E-mail: dlafaill@sec.state.vt.us
Web: www.sec.state.vt.us

VIRGINIA BOARD OF MEDICINE

Department of Health Professions; 6606 West Broad Street - Fourth Floor; Richmond, VA 23230; Phone: 804-662-9927; Phone: 804-662-9073; Fax: 804-662-9517; E-mail: medb@dhp.state.va.us Web: www.dhp.state.va.us

WASHINGTON CHIROPRACTIC QUALITY ASSURANCE COMMISSION

1300 SE Quince Street; Olympia, WA 98504-7867; Phone: 360-236-4869; Fax: 360-753-0657; E-mail: cmg0303@hub.doh.wa.gov Web: www.doh.wa.gov

WEST VIRGINIA BOARD OF CHIROPRACTIC EXAMINERS

P.O. Box 153; St. Albans, WV 25177; Phone: 304-722-1424; Fax: 304-722-1425; E-mail: cskaggs@citynet.net

WISCONSIN CHIROPRACTIC EXAMINING BOARD

1400 E. Washington Avenue; P.O. Box 8935; Madison, WI 53708; Phone: 608-266-0145; Fax: 608-261-7083;
Web: www.badger.state.wi.us/agencies/drl/Regulation/dod060.html

WYOMING STATE BOARD OF CHIROPRACTIC EXAMINERS

2020 Carey Avenue, Suite 201; Cheyenne, WY 82002; Phone: 307-777-6529; Fax: 307-777-3508; E-mail: dbridg@missc.state.wy.us
Web: www.soswy.state.wy.us/director/boards/chiro.htm

Appendix E

Chiropractic Colleges & Universities

AUSTRALIA

RMIT University Melbourne, School of Chiropractic, Osteopathy and Complementary Medicine; Plenty Road, Bundoora, Victoria 3083 Phone: 61-3-9468-2440

Macquarie University Centre for Chiropractic
Suite 222, Building E7A; N.S.W. 2109 Phone: 61-2-9850-9380

BRAZIL

Aspeur/Feevale, Rua Emillo Hauschild, 70-Villa Nova, Caixa postal 2121, Novo Hamburgo, RS-CEP 93525.180; Phone: 55-51-594-2122

CANADA

Canadian Memorial Chiropractic College, 1900 Bayview Avenue, Toronto, Ontario M4G 3E6; Phone: 416-482-2340

Université Du Québec À Trois-Rivières – School of Chiropractic; P. O. Box 500, 3351 Des Forges Blvd.; Trois-Rivieres, Quebec G9A 5H7; Phone: 819-376-5186

DENMARK

University of Southern Denmark, Campusvej 55, DK-5230 Odense M; Phone: +45 6550 2978

FRANCE

French Chiropractic Institute (Institut Franco-Européen de Chiropratique), 24 boulevard Paul Vaillant Couturier, 94200 Ivry sur Seine, Phone: 33-01-45-15-8910

JAPAN

RMIT University Chiropractic Unit – Japan, Shinbashi SD Building 4F, 6-12-7 Shinbashi, Minato ku, Tokyo 105; Phone: 81-3-3437-6907

KOREA

Hanseo University – RMIT Unit, 136-220 Jaegi-2 Dong Dongdaemoon-Ku, Seoul, Korea; Phone: 82-2-924-8723

NEW ZEALAND

NZCA School of Chiropractic, 15 Margot St, Newmarket, Auckland, NZCA School of Chiropractic, PO Box 113-044, Newmarket, Auckland; Phone: 64-9-522-5530

SOUTH AFRICA

Technikon Natal, Nattechnikon 6-20187, 953 Durban 4000; Phone: 27-31-224153

Technikon Witwatersrand, P. O. Box 17011, Doorntonetein 2028, JHB, South Africa, Phone: 27-40-62911

UNITED KINGDOM

Anglo-European College of Chiropractic, 13-15 Parkwood Road, Bournemouth, Bh5 2DF; Phone: +44(0)1202-436275 or 436-200

Mctimoney Chiropractic College, The Clock House, 22-26 Ock Street, Abingdon, Oxfordshire, OX14 5SH; Phone: +44(0)1235-523336

University of Glamorgan, School of Applied Sciences, Pontypridd, Wales, CF37 1DL; Phone: +44(0)1443-480480

University of Surrey, European Institute of Health and Medical Sciences (EIHMS), Duke of Kent Building, Guildford, Surrey, GU 2 5XT; Tel: +44(0)1483-259347

USA

Cleveland Chiropractic College – Kansas City, 6401 Rockhill Road, Kansas City, MO 64131; Phone: 816-333-8230

Cleveland Chiropractic College – Los Angeles, 590 N. Vermont Ave., Los Angeles, CA 90004; Phone: 213-660-6166

Colorado College of Chiropractic (at Marycrest International University), 3001 South Federal Blvd., Box 1126, Denver, CO 80236 Phone: 303.937.4585

Life University, School of Chiropractic, 1269 Barclay Circle, Marietta, GA 30060; Phone: 800-394-5433 (404-424-0554)

Life Chiropractic College West, P. O. Box 367 2005 Via Barrett, San Lorenzo, CA 94580; Phone: 510-276-9013

Logan College of Chiropractic, P. O. Box 1065 1851 Schoettler Road, Chesterfield, MO 63006-1065; Phone: 800-533-9210

National University of Health Sciences, 200 E. Roosevelt Road, Lombard, IL 60148; Phone: 630-629-2000

New York Chiropractic College, 2360 State Rt. 89 P. O. Box 800, Seneca Falls, NY 13148-0800, Phone: 315-568-3000

Northwestern College of Chiropractic, 2501 West 84th Street, Bloomington, MN 55431, Phone:612-888-4777

Palmer College of Chiropractic, 1000 Brady St, Davenport, IA 52803, Tel: 319-326-6000

Palmer College of Chiropractic – West, 90 East Tasman Dr, San Jose, CA 95134; Phone: 408-944-6000

Parker College of Chiropractic, 2500 Walnut Hill Lane, Dallas, TX 75229; Phone: 800-438-6932

Sherman College of Straight Chiropractic, P. O. Box 1452, Spartanburg, SC 29304; Phone: 803-578-8770

Southern California University of Health Sciences, 16200 E. Amber Valley Dr, Whittier, CA 90609; Phone: 800-221-5222 (562-902-3309)

Texas Chiropractic College, 5912 Spencer Hwy, Pasadena, TX 77505; Tel: 713-487-1170

University of Bridgeport, College of Chiropractic, 75 Linden Ave, Bridgeport, CT 06601; Phone: 203-576-4278

Western States Chiropractic College, 2900 N.E. 132nd Ave, Portland, OR 97230; Phone: 503-256-3180

Appendix F

Additional References

Abenhaim, L., & Bergeron, A. M. (1992). Twenty years of randomized clinical trials of manipulative therapy for back pain: A review. Clinical & Investigative Medicine - Medecine Clinique et Experimentale, 15 (6), 527-535.

Airaksinen, O., Hanninen, O., Kankaaupaa, M., & Taimela, S. (1999). The efficacy of active rehabilitation in chronic low back pain. Spine, 24 (10), 1034.

American Academy of Orthopedic Surgeons, North American Spine Society (1996). Clinical guideline on low back pain. Retrieved November 16, 2000 from the World Wide Web: http://www.guideline.gov/VICWS/summary.asp?guideline =000932&summary_type=bried-summary&view=briefsummary&Searchstring =back+pain

Assendelft, W. J., & Lankhorst, G. J. (1998). Effectiveness of manipulative therapy in low back pain: Systematic literature reviews and guidelines are inconclusive. National Library of Medicine. Retrieved November 5, 2000 from the World Wide Web: http://130.14.32.47/cgi- bin/VERSION_A/IGM-client?28142+detail+72

Austin, J., & Paget, J. (2000). Early management of patients with back pain. Professional Nurse, 15 (6), 399-403.

Austin, W. M. (1997). Why rehabilitative exercise? Rehab Notes. Retrieved December 1, 2000 from the World Wide Web: http://www.footlevelers.com

Baker, J. R. (1999). The 50 treatment lumbar strain. Dynamic Chiropractic. Retrieved December 13, 2000 from the World Wide Web: http://www.chiroweb.com/ archives/12/23/17.html

Barnett, A. G., Underwood, M. R., & Vickers, M. R. (1999). Effect of UK national guidelines on services to treat patients with acute low back pain: follow up questionnaire survey. British Medical Journal, 318, 918-920.

Barrett, A. J., & Breen, A. C. (2000). Adverse effects of spinal manipulation. Journal of the Royal Society of Medicine, 93, 258-259.

Bartleson, J. D. (2001). Low back pain. Current Treatment Options in Neurology, 3 (2), 159-168.

Bennett, W. I. (1990). Low back pain - the scorecard. Harvard Medical School Health Letter, Sept, 2.

Beurskeus, A. J., de Vet, H. C., Koke, A. J., Regtop, W., van der Heijden, G. J., Lindeman, E., & Knipschild, P. G. (1997). Efficacy of traction for nonspecific low back pain. 12-week and 6-month results of a randomized clinical trial. Spine, 22 (23), 2756-2762.

Birkmeyer, N. J. O., & Weinstein, J. N. (1999). Medical versus surgical treatment for low back pain: Evidence and clinical practice. Effective Clinical Practice, 2 (5), 218-227.

Bogduk, N. (1999). Evidence-based clinical guidelines for the management of acute low back pain. The Australasian Faculty of Musculoskeletal Medicine.

Bogduk, N. (1999). The neck. Bailliere's Clinical Rheumatology, 13 (2), 261-285.

Bombardier, C. (2000). Outcome assessments in the evaluation of treatment of spinal disorders. Spine, 25 (24), 3100-3103.

Bombardier, C., Hayden, J., & Beaton, D. E. (2001). Minimal clinically important difference. Low back pain: Outcome measures. The Journal of Rheumatology, 28 (2), 431-438.

Boos, N., Semmer, N., Elfering, A., Schade, V., Gal, I., & Zanetti, M. (2000). Natural history of individuals with asymptomatic disc abnormalities in magnetic resonance imaging. Spine, 25 (12), 1484-1492.

Borchgrevink, G. E., Kaasa, A., McDonagh, D., Stiles, T. C., Haraldseth, O., & Lereim, I. (1998). Acute treatment of whiplash neck sprain injuries: A randomised trial of treatment during the first 14 days after a car accident. Spine, 23 (1), 25-31.

Borkan, J., Reis, S., Werner, S., Ribak, J., & Porath, A. (1996). Guidelines for treating low back pain in primary care. The Israeli Low Back Pain Guideline Group. Harefuah, 130 (3), 145-151, 224. [Article in Hebrew].PubMed Abstract PMID: 8682388

Bronfort, G. (1999). Spinal manipulation: Current state of research and its indications. Lower Back Pain, 17 (1), 91-111.

Bryner, P. (1998). Using the Oswestry low-back pain disability questionnaire. Chiropractors Association of Australia. Retrieved November 7, 2000 from the World Wide Web: http://www.caa.com.au//features/oswestry/oswestry.htm

Burton, A. K., & Waddell, G. (1998). Clinical guidelines in the management of low back pain. Bailliere's Clinical Rheumatology, 12 (1), 17-35.

Burton, A. K., Waddell, G., Tillotson, K. M., & Summerton, N. (1999). Information and advice to patients with back pain can have a positive effect. Spine, 24 (23), 2484-2491.

Carey, T. (1998). MDs employ spinal manipulation after a short training course: Limited benefits for patients. The Back Letter, 13 (11), 123.

Cassidy, J. D. (1995). Scientific monograph of the Quebec task force on whiplash-associated disorders: Redefining "whiplash" and its management. Spine, 20 (8S), 1S-73S.

Chapman-Smith, D. A. (2000). The chiropractic profession: Its education, practice, research and future directions. West Des Moines, IA: NCMIC Group Inc.

Cherkin, D. C., Deyo, R. A., Battie, M., Street, J., & Barlow, W. (1998). A comparison of physical therapy, chiropractic manipulation, and provision of an educational booklet for the treatment of patients with low back pain. The New England Journal of Medicine, 339 (15), 1021-1029.

Cherkin, D. C., Deyo, R. A., Wheeler, K., & Ciol, M. A. (1995). Physician veiws about treating low back pain. The results of a national survey. Spine, 20 (1), 1-10.

Crim, C. (2000). Clinical practice guidelines vs actual clinical practice: The asthma paradigm. Chest, 118 (2), 62S-64S.

Croft, P. R. (1998). Outcome of low back pain in general practice. British Medical Journal, 317, 1083.

Crombez, G., Heuts, P., Lysens, R., & Vlaeyen, J. (1999). Pain-related fear is more disabling than pain itself: Evidence on the role of pain-related fear in chronic back pain disability. Pain, 80, 329.

D'Alessandro, M. P. (2000). Back pain in children: Diagnostic algorithm. Virtual Hospital. Retrieved November 7, 2000 from the World Wide Web: http://www.vh.org/Providers/Textbooks/BackPainIn Children/Algorithm.html

Deyo, R. A., Schall, M., Berwick, D. M., Nolan, T., & Carver, P. (2000). Continuous quality improvement for patients with back pain. J Gen Intern Med, 15, 647-655.

Diamond, L. H. (2000, August). Why evidence-based medicine and why now? Nelson Publishing, Inc.

Di Iorio, D., Henley, E., & Doughty, A. (2000). A survey of primary care physician practice patterns and adherence to acute low back problem guidelines.

Arch Fam Med, 9, 1015-1021. Do-it-yourself back care and repair. Mayo Clinic Women's Healthsource. (1997, Mar). Copy Editor, 1 (2), 7.

Drukteinis, A. M. (1996). The psychology of back pain: A clinical and legal handbook. Springfield, IL: Charles C. Thomas, Publisher.

Ernst, E. (1999). Massage therapy for low back pain: A systematic review. J Pain Symptom Manage, 17 (1), 65-69.

Ernst, E., & Pittler, M. H. (1999). Experts' opinions on complementary alternative therapies for low back pain. Jounral of Manipulative and Physiological Therapeutics, 22 (2), 87-90.

Ernst, E, & White, A. R. (1998). Acupuncture for back pain: A meta-analysis of randomised controlled trials. Arch Intern Med, 158 (20), 2235.

Fang, E. F., Mittman, B. S., & Weingarten, S. (1996). Use of clinical practice guidelines in managed care physician groups. Arch Fam Med, 5, 528-531.

Ferriman, A. (2000). Early x-ray for low back pain confers little benefit. British Medical Journal, 321, 1489.

Fletcher, R. H. (1998). Practice guidelines and the practice of medicine: Is it the end of clinical judgment and expertise? Boston, MA: Harvard Medical School, Department of Ambulatory Care and Prevention.

Fontanarosa, P. B., & Lundberg, G. D. (1998). Alternative medicine meets science. JAMA, 280 (18), 1618-1619.

Franke, A., Gebauer, S., Franke, K., & Brockow, T. (2000). Acupuncture massage vs Swedish massage and individual exercises vs group exercises in low back pain sufferers - a randomised controlled clinical trial in a 2 x 2 factorial design. Forsch Komplementarmed Klass Naturheilkd, 7 (6), 286.

Frankel, B., Moffet, J., Keen, S., & Jackson, D. (1999). Guidelines for low back pain: changes in GP management. Family Practice, 16 (3), 216-222.

French, S. D., Green, S., & Forbes, A. (2000). Reliability of chiropractic methods commonly used to detect manipulable lesions in patients with chronic low-back pain. Journal of Manipulative and Physiological Therapeutics, 23 (4), 231.

Fritz, J. M., & Irrgang, J. J. (2001). A comparison of a modified Oswestry low back pain disability questionnaire and the Quebec back pain disability scale. Physical Therapy, 81 (2), 776-788.

Fugh-Berman, A. (1997). Alternative medicine: What works. Baltimore: Williams & Wilkins.

Furlan, A. D., Brosseau, L., Welch, V., & Wong, J. (2000). Massage for low back pain (Cochrane Review). Cochrane Database Syst Rev, 4, CD001020.

Gatterman, M. I. (1990). Chiropractic management of spine related disorders. Baltimore: Williams & Wilkins.

Godfrey, C. M., Morgan, P. P., & Schatzker, J. (1984). A randomized trial of manipulation for low-back pain in a medical setting. Spine, 9 (3), 301-304.

Gottlieb, S. (1998). Chiropractic treatment is of limited benefit. British Medical Journal, 317, 1036.

Gross, A. R., Aker, P. D., Goldsmith, C. H., & Peloso, P. (2000). Physical medicine modalities for mechanical neck disorders (Cochrane Review). In: *The Cochrane Library, 4*. Oxford: Update Software.

Guyatt, G. H., Meade, M. O., Jaeschke, R. Z., Cook, D. J., & Haynes, R. B. (2000). Not all clinicians need to appraise evidence from scratch but all need some skills. British Medical Journal, 320, 954-955.

Hagen, E. M., Eriksen, H. R., & Ursin, H. (2000). Does early intervention with a light mobilization program reduce long-term sick leave for low back pain? Spine, 25 (15), 1973.

Haigh, R., & Clarke, A. K. (1999). Effectiveness of rehabilitation for spinal pain. Clinical Rehabilitation, 13 (suppl. 1), 63-81.

Haldeman, S., Chapman-Smith, D., & Petersen, D. M. (1993). Guidelines for chiropractic quality assurance and practice parameters: Proceedings of the Mercy center consensus conference. Gaithersburg, MD: Aspen Publishers, Inc.

Homola, S. (1999). Inside chiropractic: A physician's guide. Amherst, NY: Prometheus Books.

Hanson, D. T. (1994). Determining how much care to give and reporting patient progress. Topics in Clinical Chiropractic, 1 (4), 1-8.

Hansson, T. H., & Hansson, E. K. (2000). The effects of common medical interventions on pain, back function, and work resumption in patients with chronic low back pain: A prospective 2-year cohort study in six countries. Spine, 25 (23), 3055.

Hawk, C., Phongphua, C., Bleecker, J., Swank, L., Lopez, D., & Rubley, T. (1999). Preliminary study of the reliability of assessment procedures for indications for chiropractic adjustments of the lumbar spine. Journal of Manipulative and Physiological Therapeutics, 22 (6), 382-389.

Hayward, R. S. A., Wilson, M. C., Tunis, S. R., Bass, E. B., & Guyatt, G. (1995). Users' guides to the medical literature. VIII. How to use clinical practice guidelines. A. Are the recommendations valid? Journal of the American Medical Association, 274 (7), 570-574.

Heffner, J. E. (1998). Does evidence-based medicine help the development of clinical practice guidelines? Chest, 113 (3), 172S-178S.

Hellbruck, R. P. (1997). Medical guidelines: A valid and reliable management tool? International Journal of Health Planning and Management, 12, 51-62.

Helliwell, P., Tennant, A., & Waxman, R. (1998). Community survey of factors associated with consultation for low back pain. British Medical Journal, 317, 1564.

Henderson, D., Chapman-Smith, D., Mior, S., & Vernon, H. (1994). Clinical guidelines for chiropractic practice in Canada. Toronto, Ontario, Canada: Canadian Chiropractic Association.

Henley, E. (2000). Understanding and treating low back pain in family practice. The Journal of Family Practice, 49 (9), 793-795.

Hermoni, D., Borkan, J., Pasternak, S., Lahad, A., Van-Ralte, R., Biderman, A., & Reis, S. (2000). Doctor-patient concordance and patient initiative during episodes of low back pain. British Jounral of General Practice, 50, 809-810.

Herzog, W. (2000). Clinical biomechanics of spinal manipulation. Philadelphia: Churchill-Livingstone.

Hestboek, L., & Leboeuf-Yde, C. (2000). Are chiropractic tests for the lumbo-pelvic spine reliable and valid? A systematic critical literature review. Journal of Manipulative and Physiological Therapeutics, 23 (4), 258-275.

Hogan, M., Kelly, L., Miller, M., Nelson, B. W., O'Reilly, E., & Wegner, J. A. (1995). The clinical effects of intensive, specific exercise on chronic low back pain: A controlled study of 895 consecutive patients with 1-year follow-up. Orthopedics, 18 (10), 971-981.

Hogg-Johnson, S., Cole, D., Cote, P., & Frank, J. W. (1999). What we know about the timing and site of interventions for soft-tissue injuries of the low back, neck and upper extremity. Institute for Work and Health. 1-17.

Homola, S. (1999). Placebo effect: Favorable response to a treatment that does not result from a pharmacologic effect or other direct physical action. Inside chiropractic: A physician's guide. Amherst, NY: Prometheus Books.

Hsieh, C. Y. (2000). Back school more cost effective than manual therapies. Backletter, 15 (1), 3.

Hurwitz, B. (1995). Clinical guidelines and the law: Advice, guidance or regulation? Journal of Evaluation in Clinical Practice, 1 (1), 49-60.

Institute for Clinical Evaluative Sciences (1995). Back before you know it - The management of acute low back pain. Informed Newsletter, 1 (3). Retrieved November 7, 2000 from the World Wide Web: http://www.ices.on.ca/docs/fb /fb1390.htm

Jonsson, Egon (2000). Back pain, neck pain. Stockholm, Sweden: The Swedish Council on Technology Assessment in Health Care.

Kaegi, L. (1999). AMA clinical quality improvement forum ties it all together: From guidelines to measurement to analysis and back to guidelines. Journal on Quality Improvement, 25 (2), 95-106.

Kankaanpaa, M., Taimela, S., Airaksinen, O., & Hanninen, O. (1999). The efficacy of active rehabilitation in chronic low back pain: Effect on pain intensity, self-experienced disability, and lumbar fatigability. Spine, 24 (10) 1034-1042.

Kaptchuk, T. J., & Eisenberg, D. M. (1998). Chiropractic: Origins, controversies, and contributions. Archives of Internal Medicine, 158, 2215.

Katterhagen, G. (1996). Physician compliance with outcome-based guidelines and clinical pathways in oncology. Oncology, 10 (11), 113-121.

Kendrick, D., Fielding, K., Bentley, E., Kerslake, R., Miller, P., & Pringle, M. (2001). Radiography of the lumbar spine in primary care patients with low back pain: Randomized controlled trial. British Medical Journal, 322, 400-405.

Kjellman, G. V., Skargren, E. I., & Oberg, B. E. (1999). A critical analysis of randomised clinical trials on neck pain and treatment efficacy. A review of the literature. Scandinavian Journal of Rehabilitative Medicine, 31, 139-152.

Koes, B. W., Assendelft, W. J., van der Heijden, G. J., & Bouter, M. M. (1996). Spinal manipulation for low back pain: An updated systematic review of randomised clinical trials. Spine, 21 (24), 2860-2873.

Koes, B. W., Assendelft, W. J., van der Heijden, G. J., Bouter, L. M., & Knipschild, P. G. (1991). Spinal manipulation and mobilisation for back and neck pain: A blinded review. British Medical Journal, 303, 1298-1303.

Koes, B. W., Bouter, L. M., & van der Heijden, G. J. (1995). Methodological quality of randomized clinical trials on treatment efficacy in low back pain. Spine, 20 (2), 228-235.

Koes, B. W., Bouter, L. M., van Mameren, H., Essers, A. H. M., Verstegen, G. M. J. R., & Hofhuizen, D. M. (1992). The effectiveness of manual therapy, physiotherapy, and treatment by the general practitioner for nonspecific back and neck complaints. Spine, 17 (1), 28-35.

Kuprain, W. (1982). Physical Therapy for Sports. Philadelphia: WB Saunders Company.

Leboeuf-Yde, C., & Kyvik, K. O. (2000). Is it possible to differentiate people with or without low-back pain on the basis of tests of lumbopelvic dysfunction? Journal of Manipulative and Physiological Therapeutics, 23 (3), 160-167.

Lescoe-Long, M., & Long, M. J. (1999). Defining the utility of clinically acceptable variations in evidence-based practice guidelines for evaluation of quality improvement activities. Evaluation & the Health Professions, 22 (3), 298-325.

Levine, D. (1994). Electrical stimulation: A review of the modality for the relief of pain. Sports Medicine Update, 18-22.

Liebenson, C. (1996). Rehabilitation of the Spine. Philadelphia, PA: Williams & Wilkins.

Liebenson, C. (1999). Safe back workouts. Journal of the Neuromusculoskeletal System, 7 (1), 15-24.

Malmivaara, A., Hakkinen, U., Aro, T., Heinrichs, M. L., Koskenniemi, L., & Kuosmo, E. (1995). The treatment of acute low back pain - bed rest, exercises, or ordinary activity? The New England Journal of Medicine, 332 (6), 351-355.

Manniche, C., & Bendix T. (1998). Back pain--from the viewpoint of medical technology. Danish National Board of Health. Nordic Med, 113 (7), 230-232, 239. [Article in Danish] PubMed Abstract PMID: 9755619

May, C. R., Rose, M. J., & Johnstone, F. C. W. (2000). Dealing with doubt: How patients account for non-specific chronic low back pain. Journal of Psychosomatic Research, 49, 223-225.

Mayo Foundation for Medical Education and Research (1997). Back care - what's behind back pain and what you can do to prevent it. Medical Essay: Supplement to Mayo Clinic Health Letter.

Mayo Foundation for Medical Education and Research (1994). Back pain - guide to treatments. Medical Essay: Supplement to Mayo Clinic Health Letter, Updated Nov. 5, 1998. Retrieved January 5, 2001 from the World Wide Web: http://www.mayohealth.org/mayo/9811/htm/ backpain3.htm

McMorland, G., & Suter, E. (2000). Chiropractic management of mechanical neck and back pain: a retrospective, outcome-based analysis. Journal of Manipulative and Physiological Therapeutics, 23 (5), 307-311.

Mesa Lutheran Hospital. Aftercare Instructions - Mesa Lutheran Hospital Emergency Department, 525 W. Brown Rd., Mesa, AZ 85201 (480) 461-2701.

Mizel, D. H. (1999). Rehabilitation - a valuable consideration in acute and chronic neck and low back pain in addition to standard chiropractic management: A case study. Journal of the Canadian Chiropractic Association, 43 (1) 22-30.

Mootz, R. D., Hansen, D. T., Souza, T. A., Triano, J. J., & Wiese, B. C. (2000). Application of incremental change strategies in chiropractic and multidisciplinary clinical settings for quality improvement. Quality Management in Health Care, 8 (3), 42-64.

Nachemson, A. L. (1985). Advances in low-back pain. Clinical Orthopedics and Related Research, 200, 266-278.

Nelson, B. W., Carpenter, D. M., Dreisinger, T. E., Mitchell, M., Kelly, C. E., & Wegner, J. A. (1999). Can spinal surgery be prevented by aggressive strengthening exercises? A prospective study of cervical and lumbar patients. Archives of Physical Medicine and Rehabilitation, 80, 20-25.

Nelson, D. L. (1994). Assuring quality in the delivery of passive and active care. Topics in Clinical Chiropractic, 1 (4), 20-29.

New Zealand Guidelines Group (1996). Clinical guideline on the management of acute low back pain. Retrieved November 7, 2000 from the World Wide Web: http://www.nzgg.org.nz/library/gl_cmplete/ backpain1/full_text.cfm#contents

Nordin, M., & Campello, M. (1999). Physical therapy - exercises and the modalities: When, what and why? Neurologic Clinics of North America, 17 (1), 75-89.

NSW Therapeutic Assessment Group (Nov 1998). Guidelines for general practitioners - low back pain. Retrieved December 5, 2000 from the World Wide Web: http://www.health.nsw.gov.au

Paes, B. A., Modi, A., & Dunmore, R. (1994). Changing physicians' behavior using combined strategies and an evidence-based protocol. Archives of Pediatric Adolescent Medicine,148, 1277-1280.

Patel, A. T., & Ogle, A. A. (2000). Diagnosis and management of acute low back pain. American Family Physician, 61 (6), 1779-1786.

Petersen, D. M. (1992). The piggy banks are screaming. Dynamic Chiropractic, 10 (14), 3.

Rainville, J., Carlson, N., Polatin, P., Gatchel, R. J., & Indahl, A. (2000). Exploration of physicians' recommendations for activities in chronic low back pain. Spine, 25 (17), 2210.

Rose-Innes, A. P., & Engstrom, J. W. (1998). Low back pain: An algorithmic approach to diagnosis and management. Geriatrics, 53 (10), 26-45.

Rossignol, M., Abenhaim, L., Seguin, P., Neveu, A., Collett, J., Ducruet, T., & Shapiro, S. (2000). Coordination of primary health care for back pain: A randomized controlled trial. Spine, 25 (2), 251-259.

Royal College of General Practitioners (1997). The Back Book (3rd ed.). Norwich, UK: The Stationery Office, Lt.

Sackett, D. L. (1996). Evidence based medicine: What it is and what it isn't. British Medical Journal, 312 (7023), 71-72.

Samanta, A., & Beardsley, J. (1999). Low back pain: Which is the best way forward. British Medical Journal, 318, 1122-1123.

Sandmark, H., & Nisell, R. (1995). Validity of five common manual neck pain provoking tests. Scandinavian Journal of Rehabilitative Medicine, 27 (3), 131-136.

Scottsdale Memorial Hospital. Aftercare Instructions - Scottsdale Memorial Hospital Emergency Department, 7400 E. Osborn Rd., Scottsdale, AZ 85251 (480) 481-4810.

Serfelis, T., Nemeth, G., Carlsson, A. M., & Gillstrom, P. (1998). Conservative treatment in patients sick-listed for acute low-back pain: A prospective randomised study with 12 months' follow-up. European Spine Journal, 7 (6), 461.

Skogsbergh, D. R., & Chapman, S. A. (1994). Dealing with the chronic patient. Topics in Clinical Chiropractic, 1 (4), 9-19.

Smits, P. B. A., Verbeek, J. H. A. M., van Dijk, F. J. H., Metz, J. C. M., & ten Cate, T. J. (2000). Evaluation of a postgraduate educational programme for occupational physicians on work rehabilitation guidelines for patients with low back pain. Occupation and Environmental Medicine, 57, 645-646.

Spencer, J. W. & Jacobs, J. J. (1999). Complementary/alternative medicine: An evidence-based approach. St. Louis, MO: Mosby, Inc.

Thomas, L., Cullum, N., McColl, E., Rousseau, N., Soutter, J., & Steen, N. (2000). Guidelines in profesions allied to medicine (Cochrane Review). In: *The Cochrane Library*, Issue 4, 2000. Oxford: Update software.

Torstensen, T. A., Ljunggren, A. E., Meen, H. D., Odland, E., Jowinckel, P., & af Geijerstam, S. (1998). Efficiency and costs of medical exercise therapy, conventional physiotherapy, and self-exercise in patients with chronic low back pain: A pragmatic, randomized, single-blinded, controlled trial with 1-year follow-up. Spine, 23 (23), 2616-2624.

Toyoshima, H., Toth, P. P., & Graber, M. A. (1999). Orthopedics: Low back pain. Retrieved December 17, 2000 from the World Wide Web: http://www.vh.org/Providers/ClinRef/FPHandbook/Chapter 06/13-6.html

Twomey, L., & Taylor, J. (1995). Exercise and spinal manipulation in the treatment of low back pain. Spine, 20 (5), 615-619.

U.S. Department of Health and Human Services, Agency for Health Care Policy and Research (1994). Acute low back problems in adults. (AHCPR Publication No. 95-0642). Rockford, MD: Author.

U.S. Department of Health and Human Services, Office of the Inspector General. Federal compliance program. Retrieved January 7, 2000 from the World Wide Web: http://www.dhhs.gov/progorg/oig/new.html

van der Velde, G., & Mierau, D. (2000). The effect of exercise on percentile rank aerobic capacity, pain, and self-rated disability in patients with chronic low-back pain: A retrospective chart review. Archives of Physical Medicine and Rehabilitation, 81, 1457-1463.

van der Windt, D. A., van der Heijden, G. J., van der Berg, S. G., ter Riet, G., de Winter, A. F., & Bouter, L. M. (1999). Ultrasound therapy for musculoskeletal disorders: A systematic review. Pain, 81, 257-271.

van Tulder, M. W., Cherkin, D. C., Berman, B., Lao, L., & Koes, B. W. (2000). Acupuncture for low back pain. Cochrane Database Syst Rev, 2, CD001351.

van Tulder, M. W., Koes, B. W., & Bouter, L. M. (1997). Conservative treatment of acute and chronic nonspecific low back pain: A systematic review of randomised controlled trials of the most common interventions. Spine, 22 (18), 2128-2156.

van Tulder, M., Malmivaara, A., Esmail, R., & Koes, B. (2000). Exercise therapy for low back pain: A systematic review within the framework of the Cochrane Collaboration Review Group. Spine, 25 (21), 2784.

Vautravers, P., & Isner-Horobeti, M. E. (2000). Spinal manipulation in the treatment of common low back pain. Rev Prat, 50 (16), 1784.

Waddell, G. (1998). The back pain revolution. London: Churchill Livingstone.

Waddell, G., McIntosh, A., Hutchinson, A., Feder, G., & Lewis, M. (1996). Clinical guidelines for the management of acute low back pain. London: Royal College of General Practitioners.

Walker, B. F. (2000). The prevalence of low back pain: A systematic review of the literature from 1966 to 1998. Journal of Spine Disorders, 13 (3), 205-217.

Watkins, C., Harvey, I., Langley, C., Gray, S., & Faulkner, A. (1999). General practitioners' use of guidelines in the consultation and their attitudes to them. British Journal of General Practice, 49, 11-15.

Weinstein, S. L. (1999). Natural history. Spine, 24 (24), 2592-2600.

Wilson, I. B., Dukes, K., Greenfield, S., Kaplan, S., & Hillman, B. (2001). Patients' role in the use of radiology testing for common office practice complaints. Archives of Internal Medicine, 161 (2), 256.

Wittink, H., Michel, T. H., Kulich, R., Wagner, A., Sukiennik, A., & Rogers, W. (2000). Aerobic fitness testing in patients with chronic low back pain: Which test is best? Spine, 25 (13), 1704.

Wolff, M., Bower, D. J., Marbella, A. M., & Casanova, J. E. (1998). US family physicians' experiences with practice guidelines. Family Medicine, 30 (2), 117- 121.

Yamey, G. (2000). Can complementary medicine be evidence based? Western Journal of Medicine, 173, 4-5.

Zoega, B., Karrholm, J., & Lind, B. (2000). Outcome scores in degenerative cervical disc surgery. European Spine Journal, 9, 137-143.

Notable Quotes

"Your spinal column supports three things: your head, your neck, and your chiropractor."

~Reportedly said by D.D. Palmer, the founder of chiropractic in 1895

"If chiropractic is to thrive, numerous changes need to be made. Oh, it could continue to survive without change, like it has for the past 106+ years, the unwanted step-child of the medical profession."

~Preston Long, author.

"Hints that for an extra fifty bucks, he'll 'straighten' something else."

~David Letterman, the "Top Ten Signs You've Gone to a Bad Chiropractor" from *Late Night with David Letterman*.

"Back pain has become a major problem because there are more people making a living off this problem than dying from it."

~Reed Phillips, D.C.

"Back pain is a 20th Century medical disaster."

~Gordon Waddell, M.D.

Index

abdominal exercises, 111
acute back pain, 9, 12, 36, 39, 40, 78, 104, 126, 172
  published guidelines, 114
acute low back pain, 65, 66, 67, 68, 98, 129, 141, 142, 143, 162, 189, 193, 194, 196
adjustment, 39
  for neck pain, 11
advocate, a true, 10
Agency for Health Care Policy and Research, 65, 114, 126, 145, 147, 166, 167, 172
AHCPR, 66, 145, 146, 166, 167, 172, 195. *See* Agency for Health Care Policy and Research
AIDS, 38, 52
Alberta Medical Association, 44, 90, 170
allergens, 17, 21
allergies, 17
Alleve, 105
alphabet soup (initials), 82
Alternative Medicine and Ethics, 65, 72, 169
alternative medicine practitioners, 10, 66, 71, 75, 78, 98
American Academy of Orthopedic Surgeons, 113
anecdotal evidence
  definition of, 70
animals, 14
antigens, 21
Associated Press, 25
asthma, 42
aura adjustments, 7, 34, 44
average income of chiropractor, 16
bachelors degree
  for admittance, 15
back pain
  acute, 15
  how much of the population will suffer?, 9
  mechanical, 15
  severity, 10
back pain accompanied by nerve pain, 85
back problems
  how much of the population has them?, 6
bacterial infections, 42
Beecher
  Henry K, M.D., 54
blood work, 20, 99
brain function, 40
breach of contract, 23
bronchial tubes, 17
bruised karma, 7
C-5 fracture, 39
CAM, 101
CAM provider. *See also* complementary and alternative medicine
Canadian Stroke Consortium, 14
certification
  of some kind or another, 82
childhood ailments, 42
chiropractic
  adjustment
    definition of, 21
  philosophy, 17
chiropractic adjustment
  the premise of, 39
chiropractic adjustments, 38, 40, 45, 53, 56, 96, 132, 192
chiropractic emergency, 88
Chiropractic I.Q. Test, 11
chiropractic lobbying efforts, 15
Chiropractic Patients' Freedom of Choice Act of 2001, 132
chiropractic treatment
  very first, 14
chiropractor
  a "straight", 83
  general term for, 54
chiropractors
  appointed by the state, 47
chromosomal abnormalities, 41
chromosomal anomalies, 40
chronicity, 103, 111, 114
Cleveland Chiropractic College, 17, 18, 22, 23, 25, 26
Clinical Practice Guideline, 65, 145, 146, 147, 166, 174
colic, 42
College of Chiropractors of Alberta, 44
Columbia Hospital in Milwaukee, 16
complementary and alternative medicine, 10, 87

Craig Liebenson, 104, 113
criminal health fraud
  rate of conviction, 53
croup, 42
D.D. Palmer, 40, 79, 81, 137, 197
Dale Dauten, 5, 6, 34, 101, 128
Danish study, 14
deliver babies, 20
diabetes, 132
diagnostic triage, 102
diplomat, 43, 82
  in traditional medicine, 82
double charges, 49
Down syndrome, 41
drug-free care
  as a tactic to lure in parents, 43
Easy Rider, 20
EBM. *See* evidence-based medicine
environment for fraud and abuse, 10
episodic back pain, 65, 79
evidence-based medicine, 101
  definition of, 136
  resistance to, 11
evidence-based practitioner
  in place of "chiropractor", 54
evidence-based practitioners, 41, 102
evidence-based spinal manipulation, 53, 65, 140
expert on medical fraud, 72
false insurance claims, 52
FBI, 51, 52, 53
Four R's to Recovery, 113
fraud, 10, 23, 48, 49, 50, 51, 52, 53, 129, 133, 177
fraud investigators, 18, 50
George W. Bush, 15
grade point average
  for chiro college entry, 18
H.R. 902. *See* Chiropractic Patients' Freedom of Choice Act of 2001
HEAL, 19, 20, 175
  funding, 15
health care professional, 54, 58
  evidence-based, 60
Health Education Assistance Loan. *See* HEAL
healthcare provider fraud, 51
HIV, 38, 52
homeostatis, 111
horses, 14
human immune system, 21
hypermobility, 56
IMEs, 32, 33, 47, 136
insurance fraud cost per year, 51
International Association for the Study of Pain, 110
International Chiropractic Online Network, 41
International Chiropractic Pediatric Association, 41
International Chiropractors Association, 129, 130
Julie Bernet, 25, 29
Kansas City, 18
Kansas City Business Journal, 25
Kansas City Star, 25
lawsuits against chiropractic schools, 22
legislated profession, 132
legislative profession, the, 12
lifetime treatments, 130
live blood analysis, 45
loan defaults, 19
magic bullet, the, 38
mail fraud, 52
malpractice carriers for chiropractors, 14
manipulation, 39
Marvin Levant, M.D., 42
mastoiditis, 41
Medicare, 12, 15, 30, 49, 132
Menninger B., 25
misrepresentation, 23
Missouri, 10, 17, 18, 23, 25, 38, 52
mixer, 83
Morris M. Chiropractic College, 25
musculoskeletal pain, 102, 103, 113
musculoskeletal system, 111
NACM. *See* National Association of Chiropractic Medicine
National Association of Chiropractic Medicine, 82, 84, 177
National Center for Complementary and Alternative Medicine, 71, 72, 74, 168, 177
National Center for Health Statistics, 42
National Crime Insurance Bureau, 49
National Insurance Crime Bureau, 50, 51, 177
naturopathy, 70, 74
  definition of, 74
NCCAM. *See* National Center for Complementary and Alternative Medicine
neck locks
  tilted to one side, 21
newborns, 14

non-steroidal anti-inflammatory medication. See NSAIDs
NSAIDs, 105, 106, 113
old chiropractic families, 19
oncology, 45
Parkinson's disease, 132
passive care, 103
patients
  65 and over, 132
  care, 28, 33, 40, 54
  children, 43
  emotionally-invested, 57
  for students, 26, 27
  limited population of, 46
  misdiagnosed, 34
  participating in insureance scams, 34
  provided by the clinic, 26, 27
  recruiting, 23, 25, 28, 48
  rectal exams, 35
  skeptical, 38, 56
  whiplash, 32
pediatric chiropractic, 41
peer review, 33
philosophies, 15
physical therapist, 32, 67, 68, 131
physician
  origin of, 129
placebo effect on the therapeutic modality, 54
placebo effect, 62
placebo principle, 54, 57, 73, 87
  definition of, 54
pro-activism, 110
proper spinal manipulation, 53
prostitutes, 29, 140
pseudo-science, 11
  profitability of, 11
psychological distress, 134
psychological evaluation
  when it recommended, 79
pubic hair analysis, 37, 132
radiculopathy, 66, 149, 155
rashes, 42
requirements, 18
ride bareback, 46
short-term back and neck pain, 54
SIDS, 42
spinal manipulation, 21, 111
  definition of, 39
  how many weeks before stopping, 15
  legitimate benefits, 53
  therapeutic benefit, 54
spinal screening equipment, 24
spine
  cervical, thoracic, or lumbar, 39
staged auto accidents, 52
state board of chiropractic examiners, 53
Stephen Barrett, M.D., 72
strain, 15
stretching routine, 68
stroke, 11, 14, 37, 38, 47, 60, 77, 90, 101, 133
student loan default figures, 19
student loan defaults, 12, 15
student loans, 19
subluxation, 15
  definition of, 21
  what is it?, 15
subluxation theory, 17
Sudden Infant Death Syndrome, 42
symptoms of infection, 86
techniques
  number of different, 15
techniques used
  how many?, 9
Test Your Chiropractic I. Q., 14
testimonials from patients, 60
tetanizing, 59, 60
The Kindly Giant, 101
theosophy, 17
  chiropractic, 11
  definition of, 82
thoracic region, 21
three categories of back pain, 102
Tip O'Neill, 6
tobacco, 113
Top Ten List from Late Night With David Letterman, 12
Top Ten Signs You've Gone to a Bad Chiropractor, 13
torticollis, 21
treadmill, 68, 106, 107
tumor-like signs and symptoms, 85
US Department of Health and Human Services, 15
Veteran hospitals, 15
Veterans affairs, 12
veterinary chiropractic, 45
web sites targeting children, 41
whiplash, 32, 133
yourspine.com, 41